T0220700

Cancer
Vaccines

Cancer Vaccines

Challenges and Opportunities in Translation

Edited by

Adrian Bot
MannKind Corporation
Valencia, California, USA

Mihail Obrocea
MannKind Corporation
Paramus, New Jersey, USA

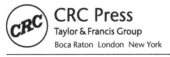

CRC Press
Taylor & Francis Group
Boca Raton London New York

CRC Press is an imprint of the
Taylor & Francis Group, an **informa** business

CRC Press
Taylor & Francis Group
6000 Broken Sound Parkway NW, Suite 300
Boca Raton, FL 33487-2742

First issued in paperback 2019

ISBN-13: 978-1-4200-5467-5 (hbk)
ISBN-13: 978-0-367-38755-6 (pbk)

This book contains information obtained from authentic and highly regarded sources. While all reasonable efforts have been made to publish reliable data and information, neither the author[s] nor the publisher can accept any legal responsibility or liability for any errors or omissions that may be made. The publishers wish to make clear that any views or opinions expressed in this book by individual editors, authors or contributors are personal to them and do not necessarily reflect the views/opinions of the publishers. The information or guidance contained in this book is intended for use by medical, scientific or health-care professionals and is provided strictly as a supplement to the medical or ot her professional's own judgement, their knowledge of the patient's medical history, relevant manufacturer's instructions and the appropriate best practice guidelines. Because of the rapid advances in medical science, any information or advice on dosages, procedures or diagnoses should be independently verified. The reader is stronglyurged to consult the relevant national drug formulary and the drug companies' and device or material manufacturers' printed instructions, and their websites, before administering or utilizing any of the drugs, devices or materials mentioned in this book. This book does not indicate whether a particular treatment is appropriate or suitable for a particular individual. Ultimately it is the sole responsibility of the medical professional to make his or her own professional judgements, so as to advise and treat patients appropriately. The authors and publishers have also attempted to trace the copyright holders of all material reproduced in this publication and apologize to copyright holders if permission to publish in this form has not been obtained. If any copyright material has not been acknowledged please write and let us know so we may rectify in any future reprint.

Library of Congress Cataloging-in-Publication Data

Cancer vaccines : challenges and opportunities in translation / edited by Adrian Bot, Mihail Obrocea.
    p. ; cm. — (Translational medicine series ; 6)
   Includes bibliographical references and index.
   ISBN-13: 978-1-4200-5467-5 (hb : alk. paper)

   ISBN-10: 1-4200-5467-8 (hb : alk. paper) 1. Cancer vaccines.
I. Bot, Adrian. II. Obrocea, Mihail. III. Series.
   [DNLM: 1. Cancer Vaccines—therapeutic use. QZ 266 C21983 2008]

   RC271.I45C42 2008

   616.99′4061—dc22

                                                        2007047354

Visit the Taylor & Francis Web site at
http://www.taylorandfrancis.com

and the CRC Press Web site at
http://www.crcpress.com

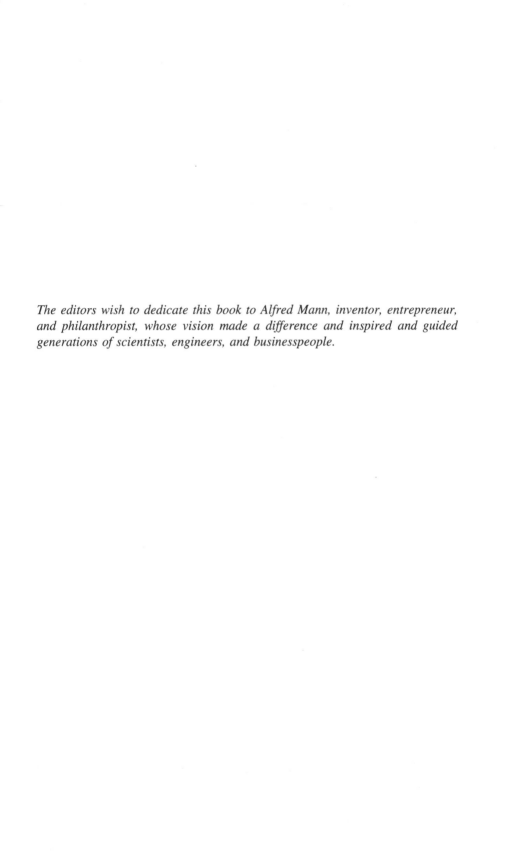

The editors wish to dedicate this book to Alfred Mann, inventor, entrepreneur, and philanthropist, whose vision made a difference and inspired and guided generations of scientists, engineers, and businesspeople.

Preface

Throughout the last 20 years, progress in the field of molecular targeted therapies and genomics resulted in significant advances in the treatment of hematological and solid tumor malignancies. Nevertheless, the holy grail of cancer therapy, to transform this illness into a manageable chronic condition or cure it altogether, remains elusive. In spite of all the therapeutic advances made recently in cancer therapy, there is still a lack of adequate therapeutic approaches to manage cancer patients over long periods using conventional treatments. Therefore, the field of cancer vaccines or immunotherapies in general may provide a ray of hope for the future. Despite sustained research and development at both preclinical and clinical stages—in academic and industry settings for over two decades—there is still no approved therapeutic cancer vaccine in the United States. Promising preclinical data in a wide range of models still remain to be translated into innovative, safe, and effective therapeutic vaccines or active immunotherapies in cancer. It is the editors' conviction that in light of the challenges associated with development of safe and effective cancer vaccines, it is more important to critically examine the failures, dissect past experience, and daringly challenge conventional paradigms that were artificially imported from other therapeutic areas of drug development. A translational approach (bench to bedside and reverse) aimed to optimize therapeutic platforms and guide the early development process to patient populations that would likely benefit most would require both significant time and financial commitment. However, this is a necessary evil for the success of not only cancer vaccines but also first-in-class molecular targeted therapies in general.

Cancer Vaccines: Challenges and Opportunities in Translation addresses a wide range of readership from basic scientists with dual interest in oncology and immunology, translational scientists, clinical researchers, industry scientists, physicians, and technicians involved in the research and development of new immunotherapies in cancer to business and project managers as well as regulatory experts within industry, academia, or government. The topic is approached from a different perspective by a panel of researchers in academia and industry involved with the development of major classes of cancer vaccines. The book outlines the gaps, challenges, and difficulties encountered in the past in conjunction with hurdles associated with translation of immunology research into clinic along with potential solutions that are currently implemented.

The excitement related to the concept of cancer vaccination fueled a broad and diverse technology base currently in early or late clinical development. This created an impression of enormous activity in the field; nevertheless, due to the complexity and specificity of each of these platforms' mechanisms of action along with the heterogeneous nature of the disease target, this assessment may be an overestimation. In fact, if one takes a critical perspective at this field, the more realistic assessment is that none of these technologies is close to be mature to yield a robust pipeline of drugs that would have the capability of making a significant impact in the current standard of cancer care. Nevertheless, we believe that far from having a pessimistic view of the field, this is rather a realistic, and in consequence, a constructive stance.

The diverse technology base of cancer vaccines under development (categorized based on the nature of technology platform, in Table 1) reflects an ongoing quest for validating the proof of concept and building on approaches that have a potential to be applied across various cancers in a more economical fashion. This explains why cell-based and highly personalized approaches lead the way in clinical development and proof of concept generation. These are followed by synthetic, "off the shelf" approaches which are becoming more realistic with recent advances in cancer genomics and target discovery and validation.

There are several key aspects that are emphasized in this book: (1) challenges presented by cancer vaccine development; (2) the relevance of preclinical models and basic science on new targets in translating new immunotherapies; (3) state of the art of current major cancer vaccines programs in development; (4) the importance of companion diagnostics and markers to the development of cancer vaccines; (5) new paradigms and models to optimize decision-making in the development of cancer vaccines; and (6) specific examples of failures and successes, along with take-home messages resulting from past experiences of developing cancer vaccines.

In the first section of this book, dedicated to basic and preclinical research, Frédéric Lévy and his collaborators provide an in-depth perspective' on the science underlying new cancer vaccine target discovery and evaluation, with an eye on tumor antigen processing, highlighting methods of optimizing current technologies in development and designing superior ones. In the subsequent chapter, Daniel L. Levey discusses preclinical models of cancer immunotherapy with emphasis on autologous (i.e., personalized) approaches along with value of these models in predicting outcomes in human disease. A critical analysis of the

Table 1 A Diverse Technology Base for Cancer Vaccines Currently in Development

Major categories	Vaccine type	Vector category	Examples/stage
Targeted to predefined antigens	Personalized	Cell based	Dendritic cells transfected with antigens (phase 3)
		Synthetic molecules	Idiotypes (phase 3)
	Off the shelf	Cell based	Allogeneic cells transfected with antigen
		Synthetic molecules	Peptides, proteins (phase 3)
		Microbial vectors	Recombinant DNA
			Replicons
			Bacteria
			Viruses
Not targeted to predefined antigens	Personalized	Cell based	Primary cell lines DC transfected with RNA pools
		Non–cell based	Tumor lysate extracts, HSP (phase 3)
	Off the shelf	Cell based	Allogeneic cells transfected with cytokines (phase 3)
		Non–cell based	Tumor/tumor cell lysates (approved in Canada[a])

Note: The technologies with investigational drugs in phase 3 development.
[a]Melacine®—melanoma tumor cell lysate.

preclinical evaluation of several approaches in a diversity of tumor settings resulted in the conclusion that extension of applicability of cancer vaccines outside the minimal residual disease status or adjuvant setting may likely require a combination-drug approach.

In the second section, dedicated to cell-based antimicrobial and personalized vaccines, Roopa Srinivasan contrasts the first prophylactic vaccine against cancer (in reality, an antiviral vaccine directed against human papillomavirus responsible for cervical carcinoma) with allogeneic cell-based therapeutic vaccines undergoing clinical development. She outlines "lessons learned" from recent challenges encountered by such vaccines in late-stage clinical development. Florentina Teofilovici and Kerry Wentworth continue by presenting an in-depth analysis of personalized, autologous cancer vaccines with emphasis on heat shock protein–based approaches currently in late-stage clinical development. Additionally, other autologous vaccine approaches are discussed. Finally, John S. Yu and his collaborators conclude this section with an exciting perspective on dendritic cell–based vaccines with particular emphasis on their applicability to neuro-oncology along with innovative combination approaches aimed to improve the clinical efficacy of cancer vaccines and chemotherapeutics alike.

In the third section of this book, with focus on antigen-based approaches, Boris Minev and Stephanie Schroter detail the science, progress, and challenges associated with development of peptide-based cancer vaccines and offer an in-depth state of the art of this dynamic field. Zhiyong Qiu and Kent A. Smith continue by outlining the advantages and shortcomings of other antigen-directed approaches such as those based on recombinant DNA vectors along with methods to enhance their potency. The editors continue by proposing a new set of paradigms in support of cancer vaccine development, with a specific focus on optimizing a recombinant DNA/peptide-based vaccination strategy. Finally, Chih-Sheng Chiang and his collaborators discuss the seminal role of companion diagnostics and biomarkers in the process of development of cancer vaccines.

By and large, beyond simply offering a snapshot of current technologies and investigational cancer vaccines in development, we intended to propose strategies for success aimed to optimize and expedite development of safe and potent cancer vaccines. Consequently, this book is different from others dedicated to cancer vaccines since it covers topics relevant to industry, translation, and development, with an eye on improving healthcare in addition to science. The overall picture stemming from our effort to synthesize the progress and challenges associated with developing cancer vaccines for clinical use can be condensed into several parameters that, if taken into account, may significantly increase the likelihood of success: (1) To make a difference in clinical outlook, the vaccine needs to be capable of mediating a very high level of immune response of appropriate quality; (2) the selection of targets needs to be rigorous to allow identification of specific molecules expressed on cells that are key to tumor progression or relapse; (3) biomarkers are critical to identifying and guiding the development and application of cancer vaccines to patients that have a competent immune system and who are more likely to respond to such agents; and (4) since current data suggest that cancer vaccines seem to be more effective in a limited disease burden, positioning their development relative to standard therapies, along with carefully defining optimal indications or combination approaches, represents a success factor of paramount importance.

In conclusion, in this postgenomic era, it is time to translate this vast scientific information and expand the healthcare benefits by adding vaccines to the large arsenal of cancer therapy in the quest of continuing to improve on the treatment and quality of life of all cancer patients.

Adrian Bot
Mihail Obrocea

Contents

Contributors

Pedro Alves Ludwig Institute for Cancer Research, Lausanne Branch, University of Lausanne, Epalinges, Switzerland

Adrian Bot MannKind Corporation, Valencia, California, U.S.A.

Suzane Brian Department of Neurosurgery, Maxine Dunitz Neurosurgical Institute, Cedars Sinai Medical Center, Los Angeles, California, U.S.A.

Javier Garcia Casado Ludwig Institute for Cancer Research, Lausanne Branch, University of Lausanne, Epalinges, Switzerland

Laurence Chapatte Ludwig Institute for Cancer Research, Lausanne Branch, University of Lausanne, Epalinges, Switzerland

Chih-Sheng Chiang Division of Translational Medicine, MannKind Corporation, Valencia, California, U.S.A.

Sara Colombetti Ludwig Institute for Cancer Research, Lausanne Branch, University of Lausanne, Epalinges, Switzerland

Jozef Janda Ludwig Institute for Cancer Research, Lausanne Branch, University of Lausanne, Epalinges, Switzerland

Nathalie Kertesz Division of Translational Medicine, MannKind Corporation, Valencia, California, U.S.A.

Frédéric Lévy Ludwig Institute for Cancer Research, Lausanne Branch, University of Lausanne, Epalinges, Switzerland

Nicole Lévy Ludwig Institute for Cancer Research, Lausanne Branch, University of Lausanne, Epalinges, Switzerland

Daniel L. Levey Antigenics Inc., New York, New York, U.S.A.

Gentao Liu Division of Hematology/Oncology, Cedars Sinai Medical Center, David Geffen School of Medicine at UCLA, Los Angeles, California, U.S.A.

Zheng Liu Division of Translational Medicine, MannKind Corporation, Valencia, California, U.S.A.

Anne Luptrawan Department of Neurosurgery, Maxine Dunitz Neurosurgical Institute, Cedars Sinai Medical Center, Los Angeles, California, U.S.A.

Boris Minev Rebecca and John Moores UCSD Cancer Center, La Jolla, California, U.S.A.

Mihail Obrocea MannKind Corporation, Paramus, New Jersey, U.S.A.

Anne-Lise Peitrequin Ludwig Institute for Cancer Research, Lausanne Branch, University of Lausanne, Epalinges, Switzerland

Zhiyong Qiu Division of Translational Medicine, MannKind Corporation, Valencia, California, U.S.A.

Stephanie Schroter Laboratory of Genetics, Salk Institute for Biological Sciences, La Jolla, California, U.S.A.

Kent A. Smith Division of Translational Medicine, MannKind Corporation, Valencia, California, U.S.A.

Roopa Srinivasan Agni Consulting Services, San Marcos, California, U.S.A.

Florentina Teofilovici Antigenics Inc., Lexington, Massachusetts, U.S.A.

Kerry Wentworth Antigenics Inc., Lexington, Massachusetts, U.S.A.

John S. Yu Department of Neurosurgery, Maxine Dunitz Neurosurgical Institute, Cedars Sinai Medical Center, Los Angeles, California, U.S.A.

TRANSLATIONAL MEDICINE SERIES

1

Factoring in Antigen Processing in Designing Antitumor T-Cell Vaccines

Frédéric Lévy, Sara Colombetti, Jozef Janda, Laurence Chapatte, Pedro Alves, Javier Garcia Casado, Nicole Lévy, and Anne-Lise Peitrequin
Ludwig Institute for Cancer Research, Lausanne Branch, University of Lausanne, Epalinges, Switzerland

INTRODUCTION

Cytolytic CD8[+] T cells are critical mediators of tumor cell lysis. Their stimulation and/or inhibition are regulated by CD4[+] T cells. CD8[+] and CD4[+] T cells recognize peptides presented at the surface of antigen-presenting cells (APCs) by MHC class I and class II molecules, respectively. These peptides are the products of antigen processing. In the context of this chapter, the term "antigen processing" defines the ensemble of biochemical pathways involved in the production of peptides associated with MHC class I and class II molecules. Even though the transport of peptides across the endoplasmic reticulum membrane by transporters associated with antigen processing (TAP) is frequently included as part of the MHC class I–restricted antigen-processing pathway, it will not be discussed here.

It is commonly assumed that antigen processing produces antigenic peptides, i.e., peptides recognized by specific T cells. This notion stems from the fact that T cells are used as readouts in experiments addressing antigen processing. However, it should be noted that the pool of antigenic peptides presented by MHC

This work was supported in part by grants from the Swiss National Funds, the Cancer Research Institute, the NCCR, the Leenaards Foundation and the Hans Altschüler Stiftung.

molecules constitutes only a small fraction of all cellular peptides binding to MHC molecules (1,2). The majority of those MHC-associated peptides are immunologically silent in that they are either ignored by T cells or unable to stimulate T cells because of tolerance. Some of them might nevertheless become targets of autoreactive T cells in the context of autoimmune diseases. Similarly, many tumor-associated peptides, which are derived from self-proteins, are not immunogenic (i.e., they do not induce T cells) but are nevertheless antigenic (i.e., they can be recognized by T cells), provided that specific CD8$^+$ T cells can be efficiently stimulated. The goal of anticancer T-cell vaccines is to activate cytolytic CD8$^+$ T cells capable of recognizing tumor-associated peptide antigens presented at the surface of tumor cells. In this chapter, the major components involved in the processing of peptide antigens by tumor cells will be summarized and the impact of antigen processing on the design of antitumor T-cell vaccines will be discussed.

THE ANTIGEN-PROCESSING MACHINERY

Because peptides are mostly produced in the course of protein degradation, the main components of the antigen-processing pathway are proteases (generally referring to enzymes degrading proteins) and peptidases (enzymes degrading peptides). The processing of antigens presented in the context of MHC class I molecules is thought to occur predominantly in the cytosol and the endoplasmic reticulum, while the processing of MHC class II–restricted antigens takes place primarily within the endo/lysosomal compartment.

Processing of MHC Class I–Restricted Peptide Antigens

20 S Proteasomes

MHC class I molecules generally bind peptides of 8 to 10 amino acids in length and present them to CD8$^+$ T cells; however, longer peptides have also been found (3). The vast majority of these peptide antigens derive from proteins degraded by the proteasomes, a multicatalytic protease complex of the cytosol and nucleus. The core unit of the proteasome, the 20 S proteasome, is composed of 2 pairs of 14 different subunits arranged in 4 heptameric rings. Each of the two outer rings contains seven α subunits (α1–α7) and each of the two inner rings contains seven β subunits (β1–β7). The catalytic activities of the proteasome are confined to the inner cavity formed by the two β rings and are associated with three pairs of particular β subunits. There are at least four types of 20 S proteasomes: the standard proteasome, the immunoproteasome, the intermediate proteasome, and the thymoproteasome (4–6). Each type differs from the others by the composition of their catalytic subunits. The standard proteasome contains the catalytic subunits β1, β2, and β5; the immunoproteasome contains the subunits β1i/LMP2, β2i/MECL1, and β5i/LMP7; the intermediate proteasome contains the subunits β1i/LMP2, β2, β5i/LMP7 or β1, β2, and β5i/LMP7; and the thymoproteasome contains the subunits β1i/LMP2, β2i/MECL1, and β5t

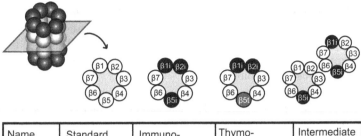

Name	Standard proteasome	Immuno-proteasome	Thymo-proteasome	Intermediate proteasomes
β subunits	β1, β2, β5	β1i, β2i, β5i	β1i, β2i, β5t	β1i, β2, β5i β1, β2, β5i
Cells	Constitutive in most cell types	Constitutive in DCs Inducible by IFN-γ in other cells	cTECs	?
Enzymatic activities	Trypsin-like Caspase-like Chymotrypsin-like	↔Trypsin-like ↓ Caspase-like ↑ Chymotrypsin-like	↓Chymotrypsin-like	?

Figure 1 Types of proteasomes.

(Fig. 1). Two transcripts of the subunit β5i/LMP7 (LMP7-E1 and LMP7-E2) have been detected in human cells (7). LMP7-E1 differs from LMP7-E2 by the usage of a different pro-sequence, an N-terminal sequence that protects the catalytic Thr residue from acetylation before completion of the assembly of the proteasome particle, and that is removed from the mature form of the subunit. Whereas LMP-E2 is normally incorporated into maturing immunoproteasomes, LMP7-E1 is not productively incorporated.

Most cells express the standard proteasome constitutively. Upon treatment with Interferon-γ (IFN-γ), type I IFNs, or TNF-α, synthesis of immunoproteasome subunits is induced (8–10). As the conversion of the proteasomes requires de novo proteasome assembly and degradation of stably assembled proteasomes [$t_{1/2} > 2$–15 days (11,12)], this process takes several days to complete. Specialized cells, such as dendritic cells (DCs), EBV-transformed B cells, and T cells, express immunoproteasomes constitutively (Ref. 13 and unpublished data). This constitutive expression is independent of IFN-γ as IFN-γ$^{-/-}$ mice, in which the expression of immunoproteasomes cannot be induced, still express immunoproteasomes constitutively (14). However, expression of STAT1, a downstream effector of the IFN-γ signaling cascade, is required. The physiological expression pattern of intermediate proteasomes is at present unknown. The thymoproteasome appears to be expressed selectively in cortical epithelial cells of the thymus (cTECs) (6). These cells have been shown to mediate the positive selection of thymocytes, a process by which thymocytes expressing a T-cell receptor with "moderate" affinity for MHC molecules survive, while those unable to recognize MHC molecules undergo apoptosis. The specific expression pattern of this type of proteasome suggests that it may play a role in the selection of the T-cell repertoire.

Even though all types of proteasomes are capable of degrading proteins, the cleavage pattern of each type is different. The standard proteasomes possess three enzymatic activities, termed caspase-like activity, trypsin-like activity, and chymotrypsin-like activity, cleaving after acidic, basic, and hydrophobic residues, respectively. The immunoproteasomes preferentially cleave after hydrophobic and basic residues but not after acidic residues. The specificities of the intermediate proteasomes have yet been reported while thymoproteasomes appear to cleave less efficiently after hydrophobic residues. These differences, while not affecting general protein turnover, have a major impact on the processing of antigens since the proteasomes are the major source of MHC class I–restricted peptide antigens. A large number of biochemical analyses has shown that the C-termini of most MHC class I ligands are produced by proteasomes (15). Inversely, peptides whose C-termini are not generated by proteasomes fail to be presented by MHC class I molecules in cells (16). This fact is explained by the absence of carboxypeptidases in the cytosol of mammalian cells. In contrast, the proteolytic production of the appropriate N-termini by the proteasome is not essential as many aminopeptidases are capable of trimming N-terminally extended proteasome products (see below). Of note, it has been recently reported that proteasomes can generate, through peptide splicing, peptides with noncontiguous amino acid sequences (17,18). The frequency of this phenomenon remains unknown, but it indicates that the diversity of proteasome products is probably larger than anticipated.

Several tumor cell lines have been shown to transcribe the genes encoding the immunoproteasome subunits constitutively. It is not clear whether this transcription results from in vitro culture conditions and if these subunits are incorporated into functional proteasomes. Most interestingly, several human cancer cells have been found to express preferentially the LMP7-E1 isoform (19). Thus, despite apparent transcription of the $\beta5i$/LMP7 subunit in tumor cells, mature proteasomes may not contain that subunit and the processing of tumor-associated antigens may be affected. Altogether, detailed knowledge of the proteasome composition of the intended target cells is important in selecting appropriate T-cell vaccines.

The PA28 Complex

The PA28 complex (or 11 S regulator) is composed of α/β heterodimers and binds to the α rings of the 20 S core (20,21). The main activity of PA28 described to date is to activate the 20 S proteasome, probably by opening the extremity of the proteasome to facilitate the access of substrates to the inner enzymatic cavities (22). However, the role of the PA28 complex in vivo is not clear as another cap, the 19 S cap, is normally attached to the 20 S core and contains subunits capable of binding and unfolding ubiquitylated substrates. Irrespective of the exact biochemical function of PA28 in vivo, PA28 expression has been shown to be important for the processing of some antigenic peptides in cells, as the generation of the melanoma-associated peptide antigen TRP2$_{360-368}$ depends solely on the expression of PA28 (23). It was recently shown that the N-terminal region flanking the antigenic peptide TRP2$_{360-368}$ conferred sensitivity to PA28 by promoting coordinated cleavages at the N- and C-termini of that peptide antigen (24).

N-Terminal Exopeptidases

The size of peptides emerging from the proteasomes ranges from 3 to over 22 amino acids in length (25). Over 60% of the proteasomal products are shorter than 8 to 9 amino acids and are therefore immunologically irrelevant as they are too short to bind MHC molecules. Approximately 15% of the proteasomal products are peptides of 8 to 9 amino acids displaying suitable anchor residues to be directly loaded onto MHC class I molecules. Longer peptides with appropriate C-terminal anchor residues have to be trimmed by N-terminal exopeptidases. Biochemical analyses of the proteasomal degradation of antigenic peptide precursors have shown that some antigenic peptides are produced only as N-terminally extended intermediates (13,26–28), while others are produced both in their optimal sizes of 9 to 10 amino acids and as N-terminally extended intermediates (16,28–30). In the latter case, it appears that the peptide produced directly by the proteasome is preferentially selected for presentation by MHC class I molecules (30).

Many cytosolic N-terminal exopeptidases have been shown to be capable of trimming the extra amino acids at the N-termini of antigenic peptide intermediates produced by the proteasomes. Tripeptidyl peptidase II (TPP II), bleomycin hydrolase, Leu aminopeptidase, puromycin-sensitive aminopeptidase, and thimet oligopeptidase have all been implicated in the trimming of antigenic peptide intermediates (31). However, it is not yet clear if individual peptidases perform unique, nonredundant functions in the trimming of particular MHC class I ligands as the genetic deletion, the chemical inhibition or the overexpression of some of these peptidases did not affect the presentation of selected CD8$^+$ T-cell epitopes (32–34). Depending on the fragment released by the proteasomes, two of these peptidases have been shown to act either sequentially or redundantly (35). It has been suggested that most MHC class I–restricted peptide intermediates produced by the proteasome as fragments longer than 15 amino acids are trimmed by TPP II (36). However, recent studies have demonstrated that the presentation of several peptide antigens by MHC class I remained unaffected in cells lacking TPP II activity, suggesting that proteasomes only rarely produce fragments longer than 15 amino acids (37,38).

By virtue of their enzymatic activities, most N-terminal exopeptidases have also a negative effect on antigen processing by trimming antigenic peptide intermediates to sizes that are too short for binding to MHC class I molecules. In some instances, inhibition of some of the peptidases has resulted in a more efficient presentation of antigenic peptides (39). Taken together, the large number of N-terminal exopeptidases and their broad enzymatic activities predict that the majority of peptides produced by the proteasomes are trimmed to sizes too short to bind MHC class I molecules long before they have had a chance of crossing the endoplasmic reticulum membrane.

Among the cytosolic peptidases described above, TPP II is the only peptidase to date that may also produce the C-termini of a limited number of MHC class I–restricted peptide antigens, albeit inefficiently. TPP II is a peptidase that habitually removes N-terminal tripeptides. However, it has also been shown to cleave polypeptides internally (40). This activity is essential for the production of an HIV-Nef-derived peptide presented by HLA-A3 and HLA-A11 (41). However, it is unclear if the latter activity of TPP II is capable of cleaving full-length proteins or rather cleaves long peptide fragments produced by other proteases. Given that Lys residues are the preferred residues for these intra-protein cleavages, MHC class I ligands containing C-terminal Lys (typically HLA-A3 and HLA-A11 ligands) may be in part processed by TPP II.

In the endoplasmic reticulum, additional aminopeptidases have been identified. These peptidases are termed ERAP or ERAAP in mice and ERAP1 and 2 in humans (42–44). Human ERAP1 and 2 form heterodimers. ERAAP was originally shown to influence the presentation of antigenic peptides, particularly those containing Pro as anchor amino acid at position 2 (45). This is explained by the inefficient translocation of Pro2-containing peptides through the TAP (46). Those peptides are probably transported as N-terminally elongated precursor and trimmed in the ER before or after binding to MHC class I molecules. Thus, human MHC alleles such as HLA-B7, -B35, -B51, -B54, -B55, -B56, and -B67 and murine H-2L^d, which preferentially select ligands with Pro2 as anchor residues, may depend more on the activity of this peptidase than other alleles. Silencing of ERAAP expression in L^d-transfected murine L cells led to a reduction of cell surface expression of L^d, confirming the importance of this peptidase in the trimming of L^d ligands (42). However, ERAAP$^{-/-}$ mice also displayed reduced H-2K^b or D^b expression at the surface of splenocytes (but not of embryonic fibroblasts) (47,48). In those mice, ERAAP was shown to affect the presentation of some H-2^b-restricted peptides but not others, while it had no impact on the cross-presentation of soluble antigens (48,49). Thus, the proteolytic activities of ERAAP are required for the processing of a larger number of antigenic peptides than just those containing Pro at position 2. As with the cytosolic exopeptidases, ERAAP activities have negative effects on antigen processing in that the trimming of N-terminally extended peptide intermediates may continue beyond the size limit for binding to MHC class I molecules (49). Recent results indicated that MHC class I molecules may bind N-terminally extended intermediates in the endoplasmic reticulum, thereby limiting the destructive effects of progressive ERAAP trimming (50). Surprisingly,

ERAAP$^{-/-}$ cells induce potent CD8$^+$ T-cell responses when transferred into wild-type syngeneic mice (51). Such phenotype was not observed in adoptively transferred splenocytes from β1i/LMP2$^{-/-}$ mice (Ref. 52 and unpublished data), even though the population of MHC class I–restricted peptides produced by wild-type splenocytes (expressing immunoproteasomes constitutively) differ from that produced by LMP2$^{-/-}$ splenocytes. The reason for this discrepancy remains to be elucidated.

In conclusion, antigen processing is prone to large modulation by intracellular proteases and peptidases. It has been estimated that only 1 peptide in 2000 synthesized proteins will eventually be presented by MHC class I molecules at the cell surface (53). Moreover, the efficiency by which different epitopes are produced from the same protein differs by as much as 10 times (54). Finally, the efficiency by which the same epitopes are produced also varies between different cell types (55). Thus, qualitative and quantitative analyses of the processing of individual target epitopes are required for the optimal selection of T-cell vaccines.

Processing of MHC Class II–Restricted Peptide Antigens

Because tumor antigen-specific CD4$^+$ T cells and Treg play a critical role in the priming of antitumor T-cell responses and the activity of antitumor T cells in situ, respectively, the presentation of tumor-associated peptide antigens by MHC class II molecules has gained more importance over the last few years. Unlike MHC class I, MHC class II molecules bind peptides of widely different length, ranging from 15 to 30 amino acids. Several molecules are involved in the processing and editing of MHC class II–restricted peptide antigens, in particular endo/lysosomal enzymes, MHC class II accessory molecules (DM and DO), and the invariant chain. It is commonly viewed that the major source of peptide antigens presented by MHC class II molecules is provided by the endo/lysosomal degradation of endocytosed or cell surface proteins. However, accumulating evidence suggests that cytoplasmic and nuclear antigens may also gain access to MHC class II by intracellular autophagy or chaperone-mediated transport (56–58). Several tumor-associated antigens expressed in the cytosol or nucleus of melanoma cells have been shown to be processed and presented by MHC class II molecules (59–62), underscoring the relevance of this cytosol-to-endosome pathway in tumor antigen recognition by CD4$^+$ T cells. Whereas the endosomal proteases have been proposed to process antigens taken up into endo/lysosomes by autophagy (63,64), proteasomes and other cytoplasmic proteases, in particular calpains, may play an important role in the processing of antigens targeted to endo/lysosomes via chaperone-mediated transport (65). However, most of the conclusions of these studies rely on the effect of protease inhibitors on antigen presentation. Thus, additional evidence will be necessary to formally demonstrate the role of cytoplasmic processing in the generation of MHC class II–restricted cytosolic antigens.

Within the endo/lysosomes, the major proteolytic enzymes are the cathepsins. Detailed analyses of several of these proteases have shown that most of them act redundantly in the context of antigen processing. Individual cathepsin-deficient mice did not display phenotypic changes in the presentation of CD4$^+$ T-cell epitopes (66,67). Cathepsin L and S differ from all the other cathepsins in that they appear to perform unique, nonredundant functions. The two cathepsins are differentially expressed. Whereas active cathepsin L is primarily expressed in cortical thymic epithelium, bone-marrow-derived APCs and macrophages, active cathepsin S is detected in DCs, activated macrophages, and B cells (68). The relevance of these cathepsins in antigen processing was demonstrated by studying the CD4$^+$ T-cell response in cathepsin L and S knockout mice. However, it is not easy to pinpoint their exact function(s) in the MHC class II–restricted antigen-processing pathway because their role in the processing of the invariant chain associated with MHC class II molecules and of bona fide peptide antigens cannot be easily dissociated. In fact, contribution of cathepsins L and S in both, the processing of invariant chain and peptide antigens, has been demonstrated.

Another endo/lysosomal protease, the asparaginyl endoprotease (AEP), has been shown to be involved in antigen processing by mediating initial cleavages of some antigenic peptide precursors, which are then further trimmed by cathepsins (69). Unlike cathepsins, the cleavage specificity of this protease is well defined as it cleaves after nonglycosylated Asn residues. AEP is involved in the initial cleavages of the MHC class II–associated invariant chain and in the cleavages of Asn-containing antigenic peptide precursors. However, the cleavage specificity of AEP is not only limited by the sole presence of Asn but also by other amino acids surrounding the cleavage site (70). The exact role of AEP in antigen processing remains unclear: while it was originally shown that AEP was required for the presentation of an MHC class II epitope from the tetanus toxin antigen (using competitive inhibitors of AEP) (69), analysis of AEP$^{-/-}$ mice has shown that it is dispensable for the presentation of several Asn-containing epitopes (71) but it is required for the proteolytic activation of several cathepsins (72). Thus, as for the cathepsins, the contribution of AEP to antigen processing may be indirect.

As with all proteases, cathepsins and AEP can both generate and destroy potential peptide antigens (73–75). The efficient presentation of given peptides is therefore dependent on the activity and specificity of the proteases. These may be influenced to some extent by the pH of the processing compartment and the conformation of the antigenic peptide precursor. In that context, it was reported that the production of two distinct MHC class II peptide antigens derived from the same protein occurred at different stages of endosomal maturation (76,77); peptides from unstructured regions were produced in early endosomes, while those derived from more structured regions were produced in late endosomes.

Thiol reductases also play an important role in the processing of MHC class II–restricted antigens as the reduction of disulphide bridges within proteins will "relax" the conformation of the protein and will probably render it more sensitive to proteolytic attack or will allow some part of it to associate with MHC class II molecules. A specialized thiol reductase, IFN-γ-inducible lysosomal thiol reductase (GILT), has been identified. GILT is constitutively expressed in MHC class II–positive cells, typically DCs, B cells, and macrophages, and has the particularity of operating at acidic pH, typical of the endo/lysosomes. In other cells, its expression is induced by IFN-γ. The relevance of GILT for the processing of some MHC class II–restricted peptide antigens, in particular those derived from peptide precursors containing disulphide bridges, was demonstrated by showing that the CD4$^+$ T-cell response against these antigens was reduced in GILT-deficient mice or cell lines (78,79). Even though tumors such as melanomas frequently express MHC class II molecules, they do not express GILT, unless treated with IFN-γ, and do not present cysteinylated MHC class II–restricted peptide antigens (80). Thus, difference in endo/lysosomal protease and thiol reductase expression patterns between professional APC and tumor cells have to be considered when incorporating tumor-antigen-specific CD4$^+$ T-cell epitopes in the vaccine.

An additional finding relevant to vaccine development is that of Unanue and colleagues who found that the same MHC class II–restricted peptide antigen is presented in different conformations depending on whether APCs are stimulated with peptide or protein (81). It appears that peptides, which are minimally folded and do not require extensive proteolytic processing, are loaded onto MHC class in early, mildly acidic endosomes, while the loading of peptides from folded proteins onto MHC class II molecules necessitate extensive low-pH-dependent proteolytic processing in late endosomes. Moreover, the conformation of the peptide loaded in late endosomes is edited by the MHC class II accessory molecule DM, which is not active in early endosomes, and selects for peptides forming stable complexes with MHC class II molecules. In contrast, the peptide loaded in early endosomes forms a more unstable association of MHC class II molecules (82). It ensues that CD4$^+$ T cells activated by peptide immunization react poorly against the same peptide antigen when it is produced from full-length protein (83). A recent study confirmed these findings in mice transgenic for a T cell receptor reacting against peptide-derived epitopes (82). Antigen conformation is not only important for activating the appropriate CD4$^+$ T cells, i.e., those capable of recognizing endogenously processed peptide antigens, but appears to be also critical in the differential recognition of tumor and normal cells by CD4$^+$ T cells. Indeed, a recent study has shown that the antigenicity of a tumor-associated MHC class II–restricted peptide was caused by the aberrant conformation of the antigen produced in the tumor cells but not in normal cells (84).

Collectively, these studies demonstrate that the enzymes involved in antigen processing and the cellular location where processing occurs play a critical role in the production of MHC class II–restricted peptides. They also suggest that the inclusion of MHC class II–restricted peptides in T-cell vaccines should be selected carefully so as to maximize the chances of inducing CD4$^+$

T cells capable of providing help for CD8$^+$ T cells at the tumor site by recognizing endogenously processed epitopes.

Impact of Adjuvants and Carriers on Antigen Processing

T-cell vaccines are generally administered in combination with so-called adjuvants, which stimulate the antigen-specific immune response. Most adjuvants activate the innate and adaptive arms of the immune system, the latter through the induction of DC maturation. Even though the key cellular receptors—the Toll-like receptors (TLR)—that bind these adjuvants have been reasonably well described (85), little is known about the processing (if any) of these adjuvants and its influence on the efficacy of T-cell vaccines.

For TLR ligands whose receptors are expressed at the cell surface such as TLR4 and TLR11, it has been demonstrated that efficient antigen presentation by MHC class II occurred when the antigen and the TLR ligand were endocytosed within the same vesicle (86,87). However, the positive effect of the TLR ligand on antigen presentation was not mediated by influencing antigen processing. Surprisingly, a recent study reported that the uptake and presentation of MHC class I–restricted antigens conjugated to ligands of TLR2 (also expressed at the plasma membrane) were independent of the expression of TLR2 (88). The reason for this discrepancy remains unknown, but one possibility could be that MHC class I– and II–restricted peptide precursors follow distinct endocytic routes toward their processing compartment (cytosol and late endosomes for MHC class I and II peptides, respectively) or that the TLR2 ligand used in the latter study binds to other TLRs.

For TLR9, which is not constitutively expressed at the cell surface, it has been reported that the uptake of antigens conjugated to the TLR9 ligand CpG and the presentation of the peptide by MHC class I molecules occur in absence of ligand-TLR interaction but that the CD8$^+$ T-cell priming by such antigen-CpG complexes required expression of TLR9 in late endosomes (88,89). These results suggest that interactions of TLRs with their ligands do not per se influence the processing and presentation of antigenic peptides but rather the induction of T-cell responses. Nevertheless, it appears that adjuvants capable of reaching late endosomes are more efficient in inducing antigen-specific T-cell responses. Interestingly, a recent report indicated that a mutation in UNC-93B, a 12-membrane spanning protein expressed in the endoplasmic reticulum, affected both TLR3, 7, and 9 signaling as well as antigen cross-presentation by MHC class I and II (90). These results suggest that cross talk between adjuvant receptors and antigen processing exists.

Aside from adjuvants, vaccines also frequently contain nonpeptidic carriers. The function of these carriers is both to protect the antigen from premature degradation and to serve as depot. Several studies have demonstrated that long-lived and acid-resistant carriers ameliorate antigen-specific responses (91–93). Newer generations of carriers aim at combining the carrier function with the adjuvant effect by decorating antigen-containing liposomes with antibodies specific for proteins expressed at the surface of DCs (94). Again, more specific targeting and increased resistance of these vaccine combinations against premature degradation should provide increased efficacy of T-cell vaccines.

SELECTION OF TARGET ANTIGENS

Given that the aim of antitumor T-cell vaccines is to induce effector $CD8^+$ T cells capable of eliminating tumor cells via the recognition of peptide-MHC class I complexes, the focus of this section will be on MHC class I ligands. Ideally, target antigens of T-cell vaccines should be derived from gene products that directly participate in tumorigenesis or that are essential for tumor survival, so as to minimize the selection of antigen-negative mutant cells. However, the most reliable technique currently used to identify potential targets of cancer vaccines does not particularly select for such gene products (Table 1). This technique, pioneered by Boon and colleagues (95), relies on the capacity of T-cell clones to recognize autologous tumor cells specifically, irrespective of the biological role of the gene product from which the MHC class I–restricted peptide is derived. Importantly, because this technique is based on the recognition

Table 1 Selection of Target Antigens

	Advantages	Disadvantages
T-cell-mediated identification	• Direct identification of CTL epitopes • Correct antigen processing	• Availability of biological material • Relevance of the identified antigens for tumorigenesis unknown
Reverse immunology	• Rapidity • Independent of available biological material • Selection of gene products relevant for tumorigenesis	• Processing of the selected antigenic peptides unknown • Reactivity of CTL unknown
Modified reverse immunology	• Rapidity • Independent of available biological material • Selection of gene products relevant for tumorigenesis • Correct antigen processing	• Reactivity of CTL unknown
Biochemical identification	• Direct identification of bona fide MHC class I ligands on tumor cells • Correct antigen processing	• Availability of biological material • Reactivity of CTL unknown

Abbreviation: CTL, cytotoxic T lymphocyte.

of tumor cells by CD8$^+$ T cells, it inherently ensures that the target peptide antigen is correctly processed by the tumor cell. It also guarantees the presence of effector T cells capable of recognizing this target antigen. A variation of this method has been used to identify CD8$^+$ T-cell epitopes derived from mutated tumor-associated antigens (96). Tumor-infiltrating lymphocytes from melanoma patients were screened for recognition of target cells expressing the HLA molecules of the patients and transfected with the mutated gene. However, these T-cell-based approaches present several technical limitations, including the need for sufficient tumor-specific lymphocytes, the capacity of T-cell clones to expand in vitro, and the need for autologous tumor cell lines. Given these limitations, other methods have been developed and implemented.

Among them, the so-called reverse immunology approach has been most frequently used. The first step of this method includes the selection of a target protein, which may be a protein directly involved in tumorigenesis (e.g., mutated p53, survivin, telomerase). Next, the target protein is analyzed for the presence of potential MHC class I ligands. This is facilitated by the extensive characterization of MHC class I ligands and the discovery of specific pairs of highly conserved amino acids, so-called anchor residues, present in the majority of peptides associated with defined MHC class I alleles. These anchor residues are specific for each MHC class I allele, mediate the binding of peptide to the MHC molecules, and are generally located at the sub-aminoterminal (i.e., position 2) and C-terminal position of the peptide. The search and predicted affinity score of peptides potentially binding to given MHC class I molecules is nowadays automated, thanks to several web-based software (e.g., http://www.syfpeithi.de/, http://www-bimas.cit.nih.gov/molbio/hla_bind/). After selection of the top candidates, peptides are generally synthesized and used to induce specific cytotoxic T lymphocytes (CTLs), which are then tested on peptide-pulsed target cells to confirm specificity and/or on cells expressing the targeted gene product. However, several peptides eliciting CTLs are inefficiently processed by tumor cells and are not presented when expressed at physiological levels (97–100). On the basis of these limitations, modified "reverse immunology" has been developed. The procedure remains similar to the one described above, except that in vitro proteasome degradation is included. Active 20 S proteasomes are easily purified and retain their original specificities in vitro. Depending on the purification scheme, 20 S proteasomes may have to be activated by adding minute amounts of SDS or purified PA28. Active proteasomes are then incubated with long synthetic peptides encompassing the antigenic peptide of interest plus several N- and C-terminal amino acids and the fragmented products are quantified by HPLC and identified by mass spectrometry (13,55). With this procedure, the processing of candidate peptides is monitored in an easily tractable manner. Several tumor-specific peptide antigens have been identified with this refined "reverse immunology" approach and have been shown to be naturally processed by tumor cells (16,101,102). This procedure can be performed with any type of

20 S proteasomes, and differential processing by standard or immunoproteasomes can be easily monitored.

A potentially interesting variation of the preceding approach is the use of partially inhibited proteasomes. A few years ago, we had shown that partial proteasome inhibition led to the presentation of the HLA-A2-restricted peptide tumor antigen MAGE-$3_{271-279}$ that was normally destroyed by the proteasome (97). Shortly thereafter, a second epitope, derived from the melanoma-associated protein TRP-2, was found to behave similarly (98). The proteasome inhibitor bortezomib (Velcade[®]) was recently introduced in cancer treatment. Similar to other proteasome inhibitors, bortezomib only blocks proteasome activities partially. Thus, it is possible that this treatment may induce the production of a series of neo-epitopes, which should be highly immunogenic since they are not produced under normal conditions. Similarly, van Hall and colleagues have isolated T cells recognizing specifically TAP-negative tumor cells or tumor cells in which proteasomes had been inactivated (103). These T cells were shown to reject injections of lethal doses of TAP-negative (but not TAP-positive) tumor cells in vivo.

Last, a pure biochemical approach can also be used. With this method, defined alleles of MHC class I expressed on tumor cells are purified by specific antibodies and the pool of peptides associated with the particular allele is identified by de novo mass spectrometry sequencing (2). The advantage of this approach is that it directly identifies bona fide MHC class I ligands presented by tumor cells and does not require preselection of any target gene product. However, it necessitates high number of cells and elaborate technical skills. More importantly, it does not predict the existence of effector T cells capable of recognizing this particular epitope. A recent example illustrates the risk of this method. An HLA-A2-restricted peptide derived from the carcinoembryonic antigen CEACAM5 was isolated and identified by the biochemical approach from colon cancer cells (104). However, this peptide was later shown to be unable to elicit CD8[+] T cells reactive against CEACAM5[+] HLA-A2[+] tumor cell lines derived from colon cancer patients (105).

In conclusion, the approaches described above present some advantages and disadvantages (Table 1). The selection of one or the other approach will be entirely based on the availability of the biological material and the technological skills of the research laboratory.

SELECTION OF VACCINES

The primary aim of developing antitumor T-cell vaccines is to induce effective cytolytic T-cell response against tumor cells. This section will focus on the contributions of antigen processing in the selection of effective T-cell vaccines, i.e., vaccines that induce tumor-reactive CD8[+] T cells. It will not discuss the impact of antigen processing on production of CD4[+] helper T-cell epitopes, mainly because of insufficient characterization of this process. As described above, several intracellular factors can influence the processing of the target epitopes. These factors should naturally be reckoned with during the development of T-cell vaccines. However, vaccines themselves can also be administered in different forms (peptides, proteins, immune complexes, DNA, RNA, etc.), which may or may not be influenced by intracellular processing and impact on their efficacies.

Minimal T-Cell Epitope

Many vaccines are based on peptides of the optimal size for binding MHC class I molecules. These peptides are generally 9 to 10 amino acids and may contain amino acid substitutions that increase binding affinities to MHC class I molecules without affecting T-cell recognition. The main advantage of this type of vaccines is that they can be immediately loaded onto MHC class I molecules expressed at the surface of DC without any processing. However, the efficacy of these vaccines may be limited by the presence of highly active proteolytic enzymes in the serum and at the surface of DC (106,107). The removal of a single amino acid at the N- or C-terminus of the peptide will immediately produce an inactive product since it will be too short to bind MHC class I molecules.

Minigenes encoding minimal T-cell epitopes are also widely used. Contrary to peptidic vaccines, minigene-based vaccines necessitate the transfer of the nucleic acids into target cells and the synthesis of the peptide. Again, the requirement for proteolytic processing is bypassed, except for the removal of the initiation Met by Met-aminopeptidase. This experimental approach leads to potent T-cell responses in vitro and in vivo. In some cases, minigenes containing N-terminal endoplasmic reticulum-targeting signal sequences have been used (108). These constructs offer two main advantages: First, the peptide antigens are directly delivered to the endoplasmic reticulum independently of TAP. Second, the peptide antigens are produced directly in their optimal sizes by removal of the signal sequence. However, such approach should be cautiously evaluated as the site selected by signal peptidase to cleave signal sequences in the endoplasmic reticulum is greatly influenced by surrounding amino acids (109). Thus, the efficiency of antigenic peptide release may be highly variable and difficult to predict.

Other methods to generate the exact amino acid sequence of the target peptide directly in the cytosol of cells have been described and rely on the co-translational cleavage of linear ubiquitin (Ub) fusions by Ub proteases. Ub is naturally synthesized as N-terminal fusion to itself or to ribosomal proteins (110). By exploiting this natural mechanism, we have generated Ub fusion plasmids into which any peptide coding sequence can be inserted at the 3' end of Ub, as long as the first codon does not code for Pro (because of inefficient release by Ub proteases). Upon translation of this fusion gene, Ub is cleaved, liberating the peptide in its final form directly in the cytosol. Variation of this method includes the addition, at the N-terminus of Ub, of a fluorescent protein such as EGFP (97). The main advantage of this method is that the expression of the minigene can be indirectly monitored by the detection of EGFP-Ub; moreover, since EGFP-Ub and the MHC class I peptide are translated from the same mRNA, the amount of each protein is equimolar and allows for the relative quantitation of peptide production by cells (30,111). Again, as for peptides, cleavage of a single amino acid at the N- or C-termini of minigene-encoded peptides eliminates their ability to associate with MHC class I molecules. It has been estimated that the fraction of minigene-encoded peptides that are eventually presented by MHC class I at the surface of cells ranges between 1 in 50 and 1 in 17,000, depending on the peptide sequence (53,111). Thus, improvements of the current methods are desirable for some peptide antigens.

DNA constructs containing linear concatenations of multiple minimal tumor-associated peptide sequences have also been produced (112,113). Each peptide within these constructs was found to be antigenic and immunogenic. However, immunodominance of one of the peptides may appear with repeated immunizations (114,115). In other cases, peptides expressed in concatenated form (but not as single minigenes) failed to elicit specific CD8$^+$ T-cell responses (116). It should be noted that the processing of these concatenated constructs may be very different from the processing of the same peptides in their natural context as the different flanking sequences will influence proteasome cleavages. Typical example is the processing and presentation of the HLA-A2-restricted MAGE-3$_{271-279}$ when expressed in concatenated constructs (114), but not when expressed in its physiological context (97). Finally, administration of concatenated peptides containing CD8$^+$ and CD4$^+$ T-cell epitopes has been tested in humans and shown to elicit CD4$^+$ but not CD8$^+$ T-cell responses (117).

Extended Peptide Sequences and Proteins

Because of the high sensitivity of minimal antigenic peptides to inactivation by exopeptidases, it has been proposed that elongated peptide sequences should confer increased resistance to proteolytic inactivation and should therefore be more efficient at producing appropriate MHC class I ligands. Immunization of mice with long synthetic peptides was indeed more potent at eliciting CD8$^+$ T-cell responses than minimal peptides (118). Given the necessity of these long peptides to be processed intracellularly by DCs, the efficiency of this process should be carefully evaluated. It should also be mentioned that the use of long peptide vaccines may inadvertently induce T cells directed against cryptic epitopes, which do not correspond to the intended target and which are not naturally presented by the tumor cells. Indeed, immunization of cancer patients with the 11-mer peptide NY-ESO-1$_{157-167}$ resulted in the induction of T cells capable of recognizing the cryptic 9-mer NY-ESO-1$_{159-167}$ (not presented by tumor cells) but not the naturally processed 9-mer NY-ESO-1$_{157-165}$ (119,120).

By extension, whole protein-based vaccines have also been used. As for extended peptides or concatenated antigens, processing of protein-based vaccines by DCs is required for the induction of CD8$^+$ T cells. In this context, it is imperative to ensure that the processing of the peptide antigen of interest is identical, or at least very similar, in DCs and tumor cells. As mentioned above, DCs express immunoproteasomes constitutively, while tumor cells do not. Thus, a vaccine may induce a very high frequency of antigen-specific T cells because of efficient processing in DCs, but these T cells may be totally ineffective in clearing tumor cells because the tumor cells expressing the standard proteasome may actually not present the same epitope. Aside from these considerations, vaccines based on proteins offer nevertheless several advantages: First, proteins may contain multiple putative peptide antigens restricted by a variety of MHC class I alleles. Second, all these peptides are expressed in the same protein context as the protein expressed in target cells. Third, protein antigens may also contain CD4$^+$ T-cell epitopes capable of eliciting CD4$^+$ T-helper cells. Last, proteins may induce antibodies that could boost the priming of specific CD8$^+$ T cells through cross-presentation of antibody-antigen immune complexes by DCs (121). Protein-based vaccines are generally administered either as purified proteins in adjuvant, antibody-protein complexes, or as nucleic acid sequences (mRNA, plasmids, or recombinant vectors). The main difference between the protein- and nucleic acid-based vaccine modalities is the initial site of processing. While proteins or antibody-protein complexes are taken up by endocytosis and initially degraded by endosomal proteases, proteins encoded by DNA and/or mRNA are processed by cytosolic proteases. However, recent evidences indicate that the priming of CD8$^+$ T cells by endocytosed proteins in DCs depended on their processing by the proteasome of DCs (122). The pathway by which endocytosed proteins reach the cytosolic proteasomes remains unknown even though some transporters located in the endoplasmic reticulum have been recently shown to influence cross-presentation by MHC class I and II (90).

An interesting correlation exists between the induction of antibodies and the CD8$^+$ T-cell responses after protein immunization (123). In general, the efficiency of CD8$^+$ T-cell priming by pure protein vaccines is rather low. In contrast, vaccination modalities incorporating protein-antibody complexes are much more efficient at inducing CD4$^+$ and CD8$^+$ T cells (124,125). Also, regions containing immunogenic CD8$^+$ T-cell epitopes may contain B-cell epitopes (126). It is therefore tempting to speculate that the binding of antibodies to antigens not only stimulates the antigen uptake by DCs but also influences antigen processing by protecting the region of the antibody epitope from premature degradation by endo/lysosomal proteases. Such effect has already been documented for MHC class II–restricted antigens (127).

Altered Peptide Ligands

Many tumor-associated peptide antigens are poorly immunogenic. At least three reasons account for this observation. First, the affinity of the peptide to MHC molecules is not sufficient to induce stable peptide-MHC complexes required for the efficient priming of T cells. Second, the T-cell repertoire against the peptide antigens may be partially tolerized or have low-intermediate avidity. Third, the peptide may be rapidly modified or degraded. To circumvent these limitations, altered peptide ligands have been developed. However, careful biochemical analyses of the impact of such modification on processing are rarely performed. All too often, it is assumed that the processing of antigens containing modified amino acids will be similar to those containing the natural sequences. One category of altered antigens includes peptides with modified anchor residues to increase affinity to MHC molecules. The natural sequence of these peptides is characterized by the presence of suboptimal anchor residues. Substitution of these residues by canonical MHC class I anchor residues dramatically increases the stability of the peptide-MHC complexes and converts most of these peptide antigens into highly immunogenic peptides. Typical examples of this category are the melanoma-associated peptide antigens Melan-A_{26-35}(A27L) (128), gp100$_{209-217}$(T210M) (129), and several peptides derived from the tyrosinase-related protein-1 (Tyrp-1) (130). Comparisons of the processing of wild-type and modified gp100 and Melan-A demonstrated that the proteasomal cleavage pattern in the region surrounding the substituted amino acid was qualitatively and quantitatively different (26,30). However, these changes did not lead to decreased presentation, probably because of the increased affinity of the modified peptides to HLA-A2. The immunogenicity of several modified peptides derived from Tyrp-1 was also significantly increased when compared to that of the natural peptides. Again, processing of the tested epitopes did not significantly impact on their immunogenicity. However, several point mutations within and outside of antigenic peptides have been shown in other contexts to alter proteolytic processing and presentation of tumor-associated peptide antigens (131–135). Thus, analyses of the impact of amino acid substitutions on the proteolytic processing of particular peptide antigens should be performed to ensure adequate processing of protein-based vaccines.

A second category of altered peptides are those capable of breaking T-cell tolerance, such as xenogeneic peptides. Such peptides have been particularly useful in inducing T-cell responses in vivo in murine models (136,137) and, more recently, in rhesus macaques (138), and in vitro in human model systems (139). In some instances, the syngeneic and xenogeneic peptide antigens differ by only one amino acid (e.g., mouse and human Melan-A peptide restricted by HLA-A2); in other instances, the difference is more important (e.g., mouse and human gp100$_{25-33}$ restricted by H-2D^b differ by three amino acids). Nevertheless, T cells elicited by xenogeneic peptide immunizations are cross-reactive against syngeneic peptides. For the two examples mentioned above, it was found that the processing of mouse and human antigens was similar (136,140,141). However, this may not be the case for all antigens (142).

Peptides that are rapidly degraded by enzymatic activities of the serum or APCs may lead to decreased immunogenicity. Chemical modifications of peptides have been reported with variable degrees of efficacy (143). In the context of the Melan-A_{26-35}/HLA-A2 epitope, we have found that the immunogenicity of chemically modified peptide in HLA-A2 transgenic mouse models was greatly diminished (unpublished data) despite increased peptide stability and capacity to stimulate specific CTLs in vitro (143).

It should be noted that $CD4^+$ T-cell tolerance can be induced by membrane-associated, secreted, or cytoplasmic self-antigens (144). Thus, similar to the high immunogenicity conferred by the use of MHC class I–restricted altered peptide ligands or xenogeneic antigens, altered or xenogeneic MHC class II–restricted peptide ligands may be more effective in stimulating $CD4^+$ helper T cells and, consequently, $CD8^+$ T-cell responses.

In conclusion, there are to date no clear demonstration that protein-based vaccines incorporating substituted amino acids within MHC-binding sequences may be less immunogenic as a consequence of incorrect processing. Given the small number of studies addressing the effects of amino acid substitutions on the processing of antigenic peptides, it is difficult to conclude that amino acid substitutions will have no impact on immunogenicity.

INDUCTION OF T-CELL RESPONSE

Impact of Processing on T-Cell Development and Repertoire

As mentioned earlier, the differential expression of proteasomes in the thymus suggests that antigen processing affects thymocyte development and, hence, peripheral T-cell repertoire. Thymoproteasome, because of its restricted expression in cTECs, will probably regulate the positive selection of thymocytes. Thymoproteasomes have been shown to produce preferentially peptides carrying C-terminal hydrophilic residues, contrary to those normally found in association with MHC class I molecules, which carry more hydrophobic C-terminal residues. Thus, it is possible that the peptides produced by thymoproteasomes have reduced affinity for MHC class I molecules. The molecular mechanism by which the reduced affinity of peptides for MHC class I influences the positive selection process remains to be uncovered. It should be noted that the positive selection of thymocytes has also been shown to be altered in $\beta 5i$/LMP7$^{-/-}$ mice (145). Since the incorporation of $\beta 5t$ and $\beta 5i$/LMP7 into proteasome particles is mutually exclusive and since $\beta 5t$ seems to be exclusively expressed in cTECs, both sets of findings are difficult to reconcile. Moreover, another study has analyzed the transcription of catalytic proteasome subunits in cTECs and has reported that the subunits $\beta 1$, $\beta 2$, and $\beta 5$ are transcribed but none of the immunoproteasome subunits, leading the authors to suggest that positive selection is mediated by peptides produced by standard proteasomes (146). Thus, the type of proteasome involved in positive selection of thymocytes still remains to be exactly determined.

The expression of immunoproteasomes by medullary thymic epithelial cells and DCs also shape the T-cell repertoire by producing MHC peptide ligands, which induce the negative selection of high avidity thymocytes (146).

This process eliminates most potentially autoreactive T cells and is of central importance for the development of tolerance to self-antigens, including those expressed by tumor cells. Analyses of the T cells of $\beta1i/LMP2^{-/-}$ mice indicated a 50% reduction in the frequency of $CD8^+$ T cells in the periphery (147). Also, the T-cell repertoire against several epitopes was drastically altered (52). Thus, the processing of antigens by immunoproteasomes in the thymus shapes the peripheral T-cell repertoire that can be mobilized by T-cell vaccines.

Impact of Processing on T-Cell Responses

It is accepted that $CD8^+$ T-cell priming and cross-priming are primarily mediated by DCs. Both priming and cross-priming of $CD8^+$ T cells depend on the processing of MHC class I–restricted antigens by the proteasomes of DCs (122). DCs exist in at least two states: the immature and mature states. Immature DCs reside in tissues, have the capacity of capturing antigens, and express both standard and immunoproteasomes. Upon stimulation, tissue-resident DCs mature and migrate to the draining lymph node. Mature DCs lose endocytic capacity, upregulate co-stimulatory molecules, process antigens efficiently, and express only immunoproteasomes. Given that some tumor-associated peptide antigens (but not all) are produced by standard proteasomes of tumors but not by immunoproteasomes of DCs, vaccines exploiting the recipients' DCs to elicit T-cell responses should primarily incorporate target antigens that are efficiently processed by both types of proteasomes. In the context of the HLA-A2-restricted peptide Melan-A_{26-35}, which is inefficiently produced by immunoproteasome, the efficacy of protein-based vaccines at eliciting specific $CD8^+$ T cells in HLA-A2 transgenic mice was low (55). In contrast, the same vaccine administered to immunoproteasome-deficient mice elicited a high frequency of specific $CD8^+$ T cells. Further analyses confirmed that the in vivo anti-Melan-A T-cell response was controlled by the proteasomal processing of DCs.

It has been shown that particular DC subsets ($CD8^+$ DCs) stimulate T cells owing to their capacities of acquiring and processing exogenous antigens (148–150). Interestingly, it was recently reported that a $CD8^+$ DC subset, which stimulated efficiently $CD8^+$ T cells and to some extent $CD4^+$ T cells, contained higher levels of several gene products involved in antigen processing (including ERAAP, cathepsins, Gilt, AEP, and cystatins) than $CD8^-$ DCs, which stimulated primarily $CD4^+$ T cells but not $CD8^+$ T cells (151). Differences in enzymes involved in antigen processing have also been documented in the context of human DCs (152). Thus, the effectiveness of protein-based antitumor T-cell vaccines is not only influenced by the type of proteasomes expressed by the DCs but also by the differential expression of a large variety of other processing enzymes.

It was originally postulated that immature DCs residing at different anatomical sites captured antigens and, upon maturation and migration to draining lymph nodes, processed and presented them to activate antigen-specific T cells

(153). In mice, studies on immune responses against viral infections have demonstrated that the subset of lymph-node-resident CD8$^+$ DCs was the major subset of DCs capable of initiating a CD8$^+$ T-cell response in vivo (154,155). Other DCs were also found to contribute to the response, most likely by capturing antigens in the periphery and transferring those to resident lymph node DCs (156,157). In contrast, it was recently shown that subcutaneous immunizations of recombinant lentiviral vectors transduced skin-derived DCs, which, after migration to the draining lymph node, initiated the T-cell response directly (158). Unfortunately, no biochemical information on the antigen-processing enzymes expressed in the different DC subsets is available. Future studies should address this issue.

CONCLUSION AND PROSPECTS

Anticancer T-cell vaccines have to fulfill at least two conditions: First, they have to stimulate cytolytic CD8$^+$ T cells and, second, they have to activate CD8$^+$ T cells capable of recognizing tumor cells. These two conditions are constrained by the available T-cell repertoire into which the vaccines will have to tap, by the efficacy of the vaccine at mobilizing this repertoire and by factors influencing antigen processing and presentation. As discussed in this chapter, antigen processing regulates the selection of thymocytes in the thymus and the T-cell repertoire in the periphery. It also controls the presentation of tumor-associated peptides by MHC molecules and, consequently, regulates both CD4$^+$ and CD8$^+$ T-cell responses. Antigen processing may produce largely different peptides depending on the environment of the tumor. Finally, induction of effective T-cell responses against peptide tumor antigens may favor the selection of antigen-negative tumor cell populations. On the basis of these considerations, it should be desirable to select T-cell vaccines with the following properties: (i) the target antigen should be important for tumor cell development; (ii) the target antigen should be efficiently processed by standard, intermediate, and immunoproteasomes; (iii) the antigenic peptide should bind MHC class I molecules with high affinity; (iv) the T-cell repertoire should not be tolerized; and (v) the antigen should be frequently expressed in tumors. The question arises: Does a target antigen fulfilling all these conditions exist? Two classes of targets come close: the first class includes all gene products containing tumor-promoting mutations, such as mutated B-Raf and N-ras, and BCR-ABL fusion region. To date no CD8$^+$ T-cell epitopes have been found for mutated B-Raf; however, a CD4$^+$ T-cell epitope has been recently described (159). An HLA-A1-restricted peptide derived from mutated N-ras has been identified using tumor-infiltrating lymphocytes of a melanoma patient (96). CTL epitopes have also been identified overlapping the BCR-ABL fusion point (160). The second class contains so-called cancer/germ-line gene products, e.g., NY-ESO-1, SSX2, and MAGEs (161). These antigens are normally expressed in spermatogonias but not in normal somatic cells. In a proportion of cancers, some of these gene products are expressed and produce immunogenic epitopes. Unfortunately, as with the other class of antigens, the expression frequency of these genes is extremely variable, both between patients and between cells within the same tumor lesion. In conclusion, it appears that the ideal target remains to be identified. Nevertheless, several potentially promising targets fulfilling the conditions listed above exist and should be entering initial phases of clinical trials.

REFERENCES

1. Hickman HD, Luis AD, Buchli R, et al. Toward a definition of self: proteomic evaluation of the class I peptide repertoire. J Immunol 2004; 172:2944–2952.
2. Barnea E, Beer I, Patoka R, et al. Analysis of endogenous peptides bound by soluble MHC class I molecules: a novel approach for identifying tumor-specific antigens. Eur J Immunol 2002; 32:213–222.
3. Burrows SR, Rossjohn J, McCluskey J. Have we cut ourselves too short in mapping CTL epitopes? Trends Immunol 2006; 27:11–16.
4. DeMartino GN, Slaughter CA. The proteasome, a novel protease regulated by multiple mechanisms. J Biol Chem 1999; 274:22123–22126.
5. Guillaume B, Chapiro J, Stroobant V, et al. Proteasome types that are intermediate between the standard proteasome and the immunoproteasome, 3rd Charité Zeuthener See Workshop: the function of the proteasome system in MHC class I antigen processing, Zeuthener See, 2007.
6. Murata S, Sasaki K, Kishimoto T, et al. Regulation of CD8$^+$ T cell development by thymus-specific proteasomes. Science 2007; 316:1349–1353.
7. Früh K, Yang Y, Arnold D, et al. Alternative exon usage and processing of the major histocompatibility complex-encoded proteasome subunits. J Biol Chem 1992; 267:22131–22140.
8. Yang Y, Waters J, Fruh K, et al. Proteasomes are regulated by interferon γ: implications for antigen processing. Proc Natl Acad Sci USA 1992; 89:4928–4932.
9. Hallermalm K, Seki K, Wei C, et al. Tumor necrosis factor-α induces coordinated changes in major histocompatibility class I presentation pathway, resulting in increased stability of class I complexes at the cell surface. Blood 2001; 98:1108–1115.
10. Shin E-C, Seifert U, Kato T, et al. Virus-induced type I IFN stimulates generation of immunoproteasomes at the site of infection. J Clin Invest 2006; 116:3006–3014.
11. Tanaka K, Ichihara A. Half-life of proteasomes (multiprotease complexes) in rat liver. Bioch Biophys Res Comm 1989; 159:1309–1315.
12. Nandi D, Woodward E, Ginsburg DB, et al. Intermediates in the formation of mouse 20S proteasomes: implications for the assembly of precursor β subunits. EMBO J 1997; 16:5363–5375.
13. Morel S, Lévy F, Burlet-Schiltz O, et al. Processing of some antigens by the standard proteasome but not by the immunoproteasome results in poor presentation by dendritic cells. Immunity 2000; 12:107–117.
14. Barton LF, Cruz M, Rangwala R, et al. Regulation of immunoproteasome subunit expression in vivo following pathogenic fungal infection. J Immunol 2002; 169:3046–3052.
15. Niedermann G. Immunological functions of the proteasome. Curr Top Microbiol Immunol 2002; 268:91–136.

16. Kessler JH, Beekman NJ, Bres-Vloemans SA, et al. Efficient identification of novel HLA-A*0201–presented cytotoxic T lymphocyte epitopes in the widely expressed tumor antigen PRAME by proteasome-mediated digestion analysis. J Exp Med 2001; 193:73–88.

17. Hanada K, Yewdell JW, Yang JC. Immune recognition of a human renal cancer antigen through post-translational protein splicing. Nature 2004; 427:252–256.

18. Vigneron N, Stroobant V, Chapiro J, et al. An antigenic peptide produced by peptide splicing in the proteasome. Science 2004; 304:587–590.

19. Heink S, Ludwig D, Kloetzel P-M, et al., IFN-γ-induced immune adaptation of the proteasome system is an accelerated and transient response. Proc Natl Acad Sci USA 2005; 102:9241–9246.

20. Mott J, Pramanik B, Moomaw C, et al. PA28, an activator of the 20 S proteasome, is composed of two nonidentical but homologous subunits. J Biol Chem 1994; 269:31466–31471.

21. Knowlton JR, Johnston SC, Whitby FG, et al. Structure of the proteasome activator REGα (PA28α). Nature 1997; 390:639–643.

22. Whitby FG, Masters EI, Kramer L, et al. Structural basis for the activation of 20S proteasomes by 11S regulators. Nature 2000; 408:115–120.

23. Sun Y, Sijts AJAM, Song M, et al. Expression of the proteasome activator PA28 rescues the presentation of a cytotoxic T lymphocyte epitope on melanoma cells. Cancer Res 2002; 62:2875–2882.

24. Textoris-Taube K, Henklein P, Pollmann S, et al. The N-terminal flanking region of the TRP2$_{360-368}$ melanoma antigen determines proteasome activator PA28 requirement for epitope liberation. J Biol Chem 2007; 282:12749–12754.

25. Kisselev AF, Akopian TN, Woo KM, et al. The sizes of peptides generated from protein by mammalian 26 and 20 S proteasomes. J Biol Chem 1999; 274:3363–3371.

26. Nagorsen D, Servis C, Levy N, et al. Proteasomal cleavage does not determine immunogenicity of gp100-derived peptides gp100$_{209-217}$ and gp100$_{209-217}$T210M. Cancer Immunol Immunother 2004; 53:817–824.

27. Stoltze L, Dick TP, Deeg M, et al. Generation of the vesicular stomatitis virus nucleoprotein cytotoxic T lymphocyte epitope requires proteasome-dependent and -independent proteolytic activities. Eur J Immunol 1998; 28:4029–4036.

28. Niedermann G, King G, Butz S, et al. The proteolytic fragments generated by vertebrate proteasomes: structural relationships to major histocompatibility complex class I binding peptides. Proc Natl Acad Sci USA 1996; 93:8572–8577.

29. Lucchiari-Hartz M, van Endert PM, Lauvau G, et al. Cytotoxic T lymphocytes epitopes of HIV-1 Nef: generation of multiple definitive major histocompatibility complex class I ligands by proteasomes. J Exp Med 2000; 191:239–252.

30. Chapatte L, Servis C, Valmori D, et al. Final antigenic Melan-A peptides produced directly by the proteasomes are preferentially selected for presentation by HLA-A*0201 in melanoma cells. J Immunol 2004; 173:6033–6040.

31. Rock KL, York IA, Goldberg AL. Post-proteasomal antigen processing for major histocompatibility complex class I presentation. Nat Immunol 2004; 5: 670–677.

32. Towne CF, York IA, Neijssen J, et al. Leucine aminopeptidase is not essential for trimming peptides in the cytosol or generating epitopes for MHC class I antigen presentation. J Immunol 2005; 175:6605–6614.

33. Wherry EJ, Golovina TN, Morrison SE, et al. Re-evaluating the generation of a "proteasome-independent" MHC class I-restricted CD8 T cell epitope. J Immunol 2006; 176:2249–2261.

34. Towne CF, York IA, Watkin LB, et al. Analysis of the role of bleomycin hydrolase in antigen presentation and the generation of CD8 T cell responses. J Immunol 2007; 178:6923–6930.

35. Lévy F, Burri L, Morel S, et al. The final N-terminal trimming of a sub-aminoterminal proline-containing HLA class I-restricted antigenic peptide in the cytosol is mediated by two peptidases. J Immunol 2002; 169:4161–4171.

36. Reits E, Neijssen J, Herberts C, et al. A major role for TPPII in trimming proteasomal degradation products for MHC class I antigen presentation. Immunity 2004; 20:495–506.

37. York IA, Bhutani N, Zendzian S, et al. Tripeptidyl peptidase II is the major peptidase needed to trim long antigenic precursors, but is not required for most MHC class I antigen presentation. J Immunol 2006; 177:1434–1443.

38. Basler M and Groettrup M. No essential role for tripeptidyl peptidase II for the processing of LCMV-derived T cell epitopes. Eur J Immunol 2007; 37: 896–904.

39. York IA, Mo AXY, Lemerise K, et al. The cytosolic endopeptidase, thimet oligopeptidase, destroys antigenic peptides and limits the extent of MHC class I antigen presentation. Immunity 2003; 18:429–440.

40. Geier E, Pfeifer G, Wilm M, et al. A giant protease with potential to substitute for some functions of the proteasome. Science 1999; 283:978–981.

41. Seifert U, Maranon C, Shmueli A, et al. An essential role for tripeptidyl peptidase in the generation of an MHC class I epitope. Nat Immunol 2003; 4:375–379.

42. Serwold T, Gonzalez F, Kim J, et al. ERAAP customizes peptides for MHC class I molecules in the endoplasmic reticulum. Nature 2002; 419:480–483.

43. Saric T, Chang S-C, Hattori A, et al. An IFN-β–induced aminopeptidase in the ER, ERAP1, trims precursors to MHC class I–presented peptides. Nat Immunol 2002; 3:1169–1176.

44. Saveanu L, Carroll O, Lindo V, et al. Concerted peptide trimming by human ERAP1 and ERAP2 aminopeptidase complexes in the endoplasmic reticulum. Nat Immunol 2005; 6:689–697.

45. Serwold T, Gaw S, Shastri N. ER aminopeptidases generate a unique pool of peptides for MHC class I molecules. Nat Immunol 2001; 2:644–651.

46. Uebel S, Kraas W, Kienle S, et al. Recognition principle of the TAP transporter disclosed by combinatorial peptide libraries. Proc Natl Acad Sci USA 1997; 94:8976–8981.

47. York IA, Brehm MA, Zendzian S, et al. Endoplasmic reticulum aminopeptidase 1 (ERAP1) trims MHC class I-presented peptides in vivo and plays an important role in immunodominance. Proc Natl Acad Sci USA 2006; 103:9202–9207.

48. Firat E, Saveanu L, Aichele P, et al. The role of endoplasmic reticulum-associated aminopeptidase 1 in immunity to infection and in cross-presentation. J Immunol 2007; 178:2241–2248.

49. York IA, Chang S-C, Saric T, et al. The ER aminopeptidase ERAP1 enhances or limits antigen presentation by trimming epitopes to 8–9 residues. Nat Immunol 2002; 3:1177–1184.

50. Kanaseki T, Blanchard N, Hammer GE, et al. ERAAP synergizes with MHC class I molecules to make the final cut in the antigenic peptide precursors in the endoplasmic reticulum. Immunity 2006; 25:795–806.

51. Hammer GE, Gonzalez F, James E, et al. In the absence of aminopeptidase ERAAP, MHC class I molecules present many unstable and highly immunogenic peptides. Nat Immunol 2007; 8:101–108.

52. Chen W, Norbury CC, Cho Y, et al. Immunoproteasomes shape immunodominance hierarchies of antiviral CD8$^+$ T cells at the levels of T cell repertoire and presentation of viral antigens. J Exp Med 2001; 193:1319–1326.

53. Princiotta MF, Finzi D, Qian S-B, et al. Quantitating protein synthesis, degradation, and endogenous antigen processing. Immunity 2003; 18:343–354.

54. Villanueva MS, Fischer P, Feen K, et al. Efficiency of MHC class I antigen processing: a quantitative analysis. Immunity 1994; 1:479–489.

55. Chapatte L, Ayyoub M, Morel S, et al. Processing of tumor-associated antigen by the proteasomes of dendritic cells controls in vivo T-cell responses. Cancer Res 2006; 66:5461–5468.

56. Dengjel J, Schoor O, Fischer R, et al. Autophagy promotes MHC class II presentation of peptides from intracellular source proteins. Proc Natl Acad Sci USA 2005; 102:7922–7927.

57. Deretic V. Autophagy as an immune defense mechanism. Curr Opin Immunol 2006; 18:375–382.

58. Schmid D, Pypaert M, Munz C. Antigen-loading compartments for major histocompatibility complex class II molecules continuously receive input from autophagosomes. Immunity 2007; 26:79–92.

59. Wang R-F, Wang X, Atwood AC, et al. Cloning genes encoding MHC class II-restricted antigens: mutated CDC27 as a tumor antigen. Science 1999; 284:1351–1354.

60. Manici S, Sturniolo T, Imro MA, et al. Melanoma cells present a MAGE-3 epitope to CD4$^+$ cytotoxic T cells in association with histocompatibility leukocyte antigen DR11. J Exp Med 1999; 189:871–876.

61. Zarour HM, Storkus WJ, Brusic V, et al. NY-ESO-1 encodes DRB1*0401-restricted epitopes recognized by melanoma-reactive CD4+ T cells. Cancer Res 2000; 60:4946–4952.

62. Jager E, Jager D, Karbach J, et al. Identification of NY-ESO-1 epitopes presented by human histocompatibility antigen (HLA)-DRB4*0101-0103 and recognized by CD4$^+$ T lymphocytes of patients with NY-ESO-1-expressing melanoma. J Exp Med 2000; 191:625–630.

63. Nimmerjahn F, Milosevic S, Behrends U, et al. Major histocompatibility complex class II-restricted presentation of a cytosolic antigen by autophagy. Eur J Immunol 2003; 33:1250–1259.

64. Paludan C, Schmid D, Landthaler M, et al. Endogenous MHC class II processing of a viral nuclear antigen after autophagy. Science 2005; 307:593–596.

65. Lich JD, Elliott JF, Blum JS. Cytoplasmic processing is a prerequisite for presentation of an endogenous antigen by major histocompatibility complex class II proteins. J Exp Med 2000; 191:1513–1524.

66. Villadangos JA, Riese RJ, Peters C, et al. Degradation of mouse invariant chain: roles of cathepsins S and D and the influence of major histocompatibility complex polymorphism. J Exp Med 1997; 186:549–560.

67. Deussing J, Roth W, Saftig P, et al. Cathepsins B and D are dispensable for major histocompatibility complex class II-mediated antigen presentation. Proc Natl Acad Sci USA 1998; 95:4516–4521.
68. Hsing LC, Rudensky AY. The lysosomal cysteine proteases in MHC class II antigen presentation. Immunol Rev 2005; 207:229–241.
69. Manoury B, Hewitt EW, Morrice N, et al. An asparaginyl endopeptidase processes a microbial antigen for class II MHC presentation. Nature 1998; 396:695–699.
70. Mathieu MA, Bogyo M, Caffrey CR, et al. Substrate specificity of schistosome versus human legumain determined by P1-P3 peptide libraries. Mol Biochem Parasitol 2002; 121:99–105.
71. Maehr R, Hang HC, Mintern JD, et al. Asparagine endopeptidase is not essential for class II MHC antigen presentation but is required for processing of cathepsin L in mice. J Immunol 2005; 174:7066–7074.
72. Shirahama-Noda K, Yamamoto A, Sugihara K, et al. Biosynthetic processing of cathepsins and lysosomal degradation are abolished in asparaginyl endopeptidase-deficient mice. J Biol Chem 2003; 278:33194–33199.
73. Hsieh C-S, de Roos P, Honey K, et al. A role for cathepsin L and cathepsin S in peptide generation for MHC class II presentation. J Immunol 2002; 168:2618–2625.
74. Manoury B, Mazzeo D, Fugger L, et al. Destructive processing by asparagine endopeptidase limits presentation of a dominant T cell epitope in MBP. Nat Immunol 2002; 3:169–174.
75. Moss CX, Villadangos JA, Colin Watts C. Destructive potential of the aspartyl protease cathepsin D in MHC class II-restricted antigen processing. Eur J Immunol 2005; 35:3442–3451.
76. Musson JA, Walker N, Flick-Smith H, et al. Differential processing of CD4 T-cell epitopes from the protective antigen of *Bacillus anthracis*. J Biol Chem 2003; 278:52425–52431.
77. Musson JA, Morton M, Walker N, et al. Sequential proteolytic processing of the capsular Caf1 antigen of *Yersinia pestis* for major histocompatibility complex class II-restricted presentation to T lymphocytes. J Biol Chem 2006; 281:26129–26135.
78. Maric M, Arunachalam B, Phan UT, et al. Defective antigen processing in GILT-free mice. Science 2001; 294:1361–1365.
79. Hastings KT, Lackman RL, Cresswell P. Functional requirements for the lysosomal thiol reductase GILT in MHC class II-restricted antigen processing. J Immunol 2006; 177:8569–8577.
80. Haque MA, Li P, Jackson SK, et al. Absence of γ-Interferon-inducible lysosomal thiol reductase in melanomas disrupts T cell recognition of select immunodominant epitopes. J Exp Med 2002; 195:1267–1277.
81. Lovitch SB, Unanue ER. Conformational isomers of a peptide-class II major histocompatibility complex. Immunol Rev 2005; 207:293–313.
82. Lovitch SB, Esparza TJ, Schweitzer G, et al. Activation of type B T cells after protein immunization reveals novel pathways of in vivo presentation of peptides. J Immunol 2007; 178:122–133.
83. Viner N, Nelson C, Unanue E. Identification of a major I-E^k-restricted determinant of hen egg lysozyme: limitations of lymph node proliferation studies in defining immunodominance and crypticity. Proc Natl Acad Sci USA 1995; 92:2214–2218.

84. Mimura Y, Mimura-Kimura Y, Doores K, et al. Folding of an MHC class II-restricted tumor antigen controls its antigenicity via MHC-guided processing. Proc Natl Acad Sci USA 2007; 104:5983–5988.
85. Takeda K, Kaisho T, Akira S. Toll-like receptors. Annu Rev Immunol 2003; 21:335–376.
86. Blander JM, Medzhitov R. Toll-dependent selection of microbial antigens for presentation by dendritic cells. Nature 2006; 440:808–812.
87. Yarovinsky F, Kanzler H, Hieny S, et al. Toll-like receptor recognition regulates immunodominance in an antimicrobial $CD4^+$ T cell response. Immunity 2006; 25:655–664.
88. Khan S, Bijker MS, Weterings JJ, et al. Distinct uptake mechanisms but similar intracellular processing of two different toll-like receptor ligand-peptide conjugates in dendritic cells. J Biol Chem 2007; 282:21145–21159.
89. Heit A, Maurer T, Hochrein H, et al. Cutting Edge: Toll-like receptor 9 expression is not required for CpG DNA-aided cross-presentation of DNA-conjugated antigens but essential for cross-priming of CD8 T cells. J Immunol 2003; 170: 2802–2805.
90. Tabeta K, Hoebe K, Janssen EM, et al. The Unc93b1 mutation 3d disrupts exogenous antigen presentation and signaling via Toll-like receptors 3, 7 and 9. Nat Immunol 2006; 7:156–164.
91. Harding CV, Collins DS, Slot JW, et al. Liposome-encapsulated antigens are processed in lysosomes, recycled, and presented to T cells. Cell 1991; 64:393–401.
92. Wang C, Ge Q, Ting D, et al. Molecularly engineered poly(ortho ester) microspheres for enhanced delivery of DNA vaccines. Nat Mater 2004; 3:190–196.
93. Reddy ST, Swartz MA, Hubbell JA. Targeting dendritic cells with biomaterials: developing the next generation of vaccines. Trends Immunol 2006; 27:573–579.
94. Altin JG, van Broekhoven CL, Parish CR. Targeting dendritic cells with antigen-containing liposomes: antitumour immunity. Expert Opin. Biol. Ther. 2004; 4: 1735–1747.
95. van der Bruggen P, Traversari C, Chomez P, et al. A gene encoding an antigen recognized by cytolytic T lymphocytes on a human melanoma. Science 1991; 254:1643–1647.
96. Linard B, Bezieau S, Benlalam H, et al. A ras-mutated peptide targeted by CTL infiltrating a human melanoma lesion. J Immunol 2002; 168:4802–4808.
97. Valmori D, Gileadi U, Servis C, et al. Modulation of proteasomal activity required for the generation of a CTL-defined peptide derived from the tumor antigen MAGE-3. J Exp Med 1999; 189:895–905.
98. Noppen C, Lévy F, Burri L, et al. Naturally processed and concealed HLA-A2.1 restricted epitopes from tumor associated antigen tyrosinase-related protein-2. Int J Cancer 2000; 87:241–246.
99. Ayyoub M, Migliaccio M, Guillaume P, et al. Lack of tumor recognition by hTERT peptide 540-548 specific $CD8^+$ T cells from melanoma patients reveals inefficient antigen processing. Eur J Immunol 2001; 31:2642–2651.
100. Parkhurst MR, Riley JP, Igarashi T, et al. Immunization of patients with the hTERT:540–548 peptide induces peptide-reactive T lymphocytes that do not recognize tumors endogenously expressing telomerase. Clin Cancer Res 2004; 10:4688–4698.

101. Ayyoub M, Hesdorffer CS, Montes M, et al. An immunodominant SSX-2-derived epitope recognized by CD4+ T cells in association with HLA-DR. J Clin Invest 2004; 113:1225–1233.
102. Valmori D, Levy F, Godefroy E, et al. Epitope clustering in regions undergoing efficient proteasomal processing defines immunodominant CTL regions of a tumor antigen. Clin Immunol 2007; 122:163–172.
103. van Hall T, Wolpert EZ, van Veelen P, et al. Selective cytotoxic T-lymphocyte targeting of tumor immune escape variants. Nat Med 2006; 12:417–424.
104. Schirle M, Keilholz W, Weber B, et al. Identification of tumor-associated MHC class I ligands by a novel T cell-independent approach. Eur J Immunol 2000; 30:2216–2225.
105. Alves P, Viatte S, Fagerberg T, et al. Immunogenicity of the carcinoembryonic antigen derived peptide 694 in HLA-A2 healthy donors and colorectal carcinoma patients. Cancer Immunol Immunother 2007; 56:1795–1805.
106. Falo LD, Colarusso LJ, Benacerraf B, et al. Serum proteases alter the antigenicity of peptides presented by class I major histocompatibility complex molecules. Proc Natl Acad Sci USA 1992; 89:8347–8350.
107. Amoscato AA, Prenovitz DA, Lotze MT. Rapid extracellular degradation of synthetic class I peptides by human dendritic cells. J Immunol 1998; 161:4023–4032.
108. Bacik I, Cox JH, Anderson R, et al. TAP (transporter associated with antigen processing)-independent presentation of endogenously synthesized peptides is enhanced by endoplasmic reticulum insertion sequences located at the amino- but not carboxyl-terminus of the peptide. J Immunol 1994; 152:381–387.
109. Martoglio B, Dobberstein B. Signal sequences: more than just greasy peptides. Trends Cell Biol 1998; 8:410–415.
110. Finley D, Bartel B, Varshavsky A. The tails of ubiquitin precursors are ribosomal proteins whose fusion to ubiquitin facilitates ribosome biogenesis. Nature 1989; 338:394–401.
111. Fruci D, Lauvau G, Saveanu L, et al. Quantifying recruitment of cytosolic peptides for HLA class I presentation: impact of TAP transport. J Immunol 2003; 170:2977–2984.
112. Toes REM, Hoeben RC, van der Voort EIH, et al. Protective anti-tumor immunity induced by vaccination with recombinant adenoviruses encoding multiple tumor-associated cytotoxic T lymphocyte epitopes in a string-of-beads fashion. Proc Natl Acad Sci USA 1997; 94:14660–14665.
113. Mateo L, Gardner J, Chen Q, et al. An HLA-A2 polyepitope vaccine for melanoma immunotherapy. J Immunol 1999; 163:4058–4063.
114. Smith SG, Patel PM, Porte J, et al. Human dendritic cells genetically engineered to express a melanoma polyepitope DNA vaccine induce multiple cytotoxic T-cell responses. Clin Cancer Res 2001; 7:4253–4261.
115. Palmowski MJ, Choi EM-L, Hermans IF, et al. Competition between CTL narrows the immune response induced by prime-boost vaccination protocols. J Immunol 2002; 168:4391–4398.
116. Tine JA, Firat H, Payne A, et al. Enhanced multiepitope-based vaccines elicit CD8[+] cytotoxic T cells against both immunodominant and cryptic epitopes. Vaccine 2005; 23:1085–1091.
117. Slingluff CL Jr., Yamshchikov G, Neese P, et al. Phase I trial of a melanoma vaccine with gp100$_{280-288}$ peptide and tetanus helper peptide in adjuvant: immunologic and clinical outcomes. Clin Cancer Res 2001; 7:3012–3024.

118. Zwaveling S, Mota SCF, Nouta J, et al. Established human papillomavirus type 16-expressing tumors are effectively eradicated following vaccination with long peptides. J Immunol 2002; 169:350–358.

119. Gnjatic S, Jager E, Chen W, et al. CD8$^+$ T cell responses against a dominant cryptic HLA-A2 epitope after NY-ESO-1 peptide immunization of cancer patients. Proc Natl Acad Sci USA 2002; 99:11813–11818.

120. Dutoit V, Taub RN, Papadopoulos KP, et al. Multiepitope CD8$^+$ T cell response to a NY-ESO-1 peptide vaccine results in imprecise tumor targeting. J Clin Invest 2002; 110:1813–1822.

121. Nagata Y, Ono S, Matsuo M, et al. Differential presentation of a soluble exogenous tumor antigen, NY-ESO-1, by distinct human dendritic cell populations. Proc Natl Acad Sci USA 2002; 99:10629–10634.

122. Norbury CC, Basta S, Donohue KB, et al. CD8$^+$ T cell cross-priming via transfer of proteasome substrates. Science 2004; 304:1318–1321.

123. Valmori D, Souleimanian NE, Tosello V, et al. Vaccination with NY-ESO-1 protein and CpG in Montanide induces integrated antibody/Th1 responses and CD8 T cells through cross-priming. Proc Natl Acad Sci USA 2007; 104:8947–8952.

124. Rafiq K, Bergtold A, Clynes R. Immune complex-mediated antigen presentation induces tumor immunity. J Clin Invest 2002; 110:71–79.

125. Schuurhuis DH, van Montfoort N, Ioan-Facsinay A, et al. Immune complex-loaded dendritic cells are superior to soluble immune complexes as antitumor vaccine. J Immunol 2006; 176:4573–4580.

126. Sweetser M, Braciale V, Braciale T. Class I major histocompatibility complex-restricted T lymphocyte recognition of the influenza hemagglutinin. Overlap between class I cytotoxic T lymphocytes and antibody sites. J Exp Med 1989; 170: 1357–1368.

127. Simitsek P, Campbell D, Lanzavecchia A, et al. Modulation of antigen processing by bound antibodies can boost or suppress class II major histocompatibility complex presentation of different T cell determinants. J Exp Med 1995; 181:1957–1963.

128. Valmori D, Fonteneau J-F, Lizana CM, et al. Enhanced generation of specific tumor-reactive CTL in vitro by selected Melan-A/MART-1 immunodominant peptide analogues. J Immunol 1998; 160:1750–1758.

129. Irvine KR, Parkhurst MR, Shulman EP, et al. Recombinant virus vaccination against "self" antigens using anchor-fixed immunogens. Cancer Res 1999; 59: 2536–2540.

130. Guevara-Patino JA, Engelhorn ME, Turk MJ, et al. Optimization of a self antigen for presentation of multiple epitopes in cancer immunity. J Clin Invest 2006; 116:1382–1390.

131. Miconnet I, Servis C, Cerottini J-C, et al. Amino acid identity and/or position determine the proteasomal cleavage of the HLA-A*0201-restricted peptide tumor antigen MAGE-3$_{271-279}$. J Biol Chem 2000; 275:26892–26897.

132. Beekman NJ, van Veelen PA, van Hall T, et al. Abrogation of CTL epitope processing by single amino acid substitution flanking the C-terminal proteasome cleavage site. J Immunol 2000; 164:1898–1905.

133. Ossendorp F, Eggers M, Neisig A, et al. A single residue exchange within a viral CTL epitope alters proteasome-mediated degradation resulting in lack of antigen presentation. Immunity 1996; 5:115–124.

134. Theobald M, Ruppert T, Kuckelkorn U, et al. The sequence alteration associated with a mutational hotspot in p53 protects cells from lysis by cytotoxic T lymphocytes specific for a flanking peptide epitope. J Exp Med 1998; 188:1017–1028.

135. Spierings E, Brickner AG, Caldwell JA, et al. The minor histocompatibility antigen HA-3 arises from differential proteasome-mediated cleavage of the lymphoid blast crisis (Lbc) oncoprotein. Blood 2003; 102:621–629.

136. Colombetti S, Fagerberg T, Baumgärtner P, et al. Impact of orthologous Melan-A peptide immunization on the anti-self Melan-A/HLA-A2 T cell cross-reactivity. J Immunol 2006; 176:6560–6567.

137. Srinivasan R, Wolchok J. Tumor antigens for cancer immunotherapy: therapeutic potential of xenogeneic DNA vaccines. J Transl Med 2004; 2:12–24.

138. Elia L, Mennuni C, Storto M, et al. Genetic vaccines against Ep-CAM break tolerance to self in a limited subset of subjects: initial identification of predictive biomarkers. Eur J Immunol 2006; 36:1337–1349.

139. Hu B, Wei Y-q, Tian L, et al. Human T lymphocyte responses against lung cancer induced by recombinant truncated mouse EGFR. Cancer Immunol Immunother 2006; 55:386–393.

140. Overwijk WW, Tsung A, Irvine KR, et al. gp100/pmel 17 is a murine tumor rejection antigen: induction of "self"-reactive, tumoricidal T cells using high-affinity, altered peptide ligand. J Exp Med 1998; 188:277–286.

141. Gold JS, Ferrone CR, Guevara-Patino JA, et al. A single heteroclitic epitope determines cancer immunity after xenogeneic DNA immunization against a tumor differentiation antigen. J Immunol 2003; 170:5188–5194.

142. Sesma L, Alvarez I, Marcilla M, et al. Species-specific differences in proteasomal processing and tapasin-mediated loading influence peptide presentation by HLA-B27 in murine cells. J Biol Chem 2003; 278:46461–46472.

143. Blanchet J-S, Valmori D, Dufau I, et al. A new generation of Melan-A/MART-1 peptides that fulfill both increased immunogenicity and high resistance to biodegradation: implication for molecular anti-melanoma immunotherapy. J Immunol 2001; 167:5852–5861.

144. Oehen S, Feng L, Xia Y, et al. Antigen compartmentation and T helper cell tolerance induction. J Exp Med 1996; 183:2617–2626.

145. Osterloh P, Linkemann K, Tenzer S, et al. Proteasomes shape the repertoire of T cells participating in antigen-specific immune responses. Proc. Natl Acad Sci USA 2006; 103:5042–5047.

146. Nil A, Firat E, Sobek V, et al. Expression of housekeeping and immunoproteasome subunit genes is differentially regulated in positively and negatively selecting thymic stroma subsets. Eur J Immunol 2004; 34:2681–2689.

147. Van Kaer L, Ashton-Rickardt PG, Eichelberger M, et al. Altered peptidase and viral-specific T cell response in LMP2 mutant mice. Immunity 1994; 1:533–541.

148. den Haan JMM, Lehar SM, Bevan MJ. CD8$^+$ but not CD8$^-$ dendritic cells cross-prime cytotoxic T cells in vivo. J Exp Med 2000; 192:1685–1696.

149. Pooley JL, Heath WR, Shortman K. Intravenous soluble antigen is presented to CD4 T cells by CD8$^-$ dendritic cells, but cross-presented to CD8 T cells by CD8$^+$ dendritic cells. J Immunol 2001; 166:5327–5330.

150. Schnorrer P, Behrens GMN, Wilson NS, et al. The dominant role of CD8$^+$ dendritic cells in cross-presentation is not dictated by antigen capture. Proc Natl Acad Sci USA 2006; 103:10729–10734.

151. Dudziak D, Kamphorst AO, Heidkamp GF, et al. Differential antigen processing by dendritic cell subsets in vivo. Science 2007; 315:107–111.

152. Burster T, Beck A, Tolosa E, et al. Differential processing of autoantigens in lysosomes from human monocyte-derived and peripheral blood dendritic cells. J Immunol 2005; 175:5940–5949.

153. Banchereau J, Briere F, Caux C, et al. Immunobiology of dendritic cells. Annu Rev Immunol 2000; 18:767–811.

154. Allan RS, Smith CM, Belz GT, et al. Epidermal viral immunity induced by CD8α$^+$ dendritic cells but not by Langerhans cells. Science 2003; 301:1925–1928.

155. Belz GT, Smith CM, Kleinert L, et al. Distinct migrating and nonmigrating dendritic cell populations are involved in MHC class I-restricted antigen presentation after lung infection with virus. Proc Natl Acad Sci USA 2004; 101:8670–8675.

156. Inaba K, Turley S, Yamaide F, et al. Efficient presentation of phagocytosed cellular fragments on the major histocompatibility complex class II products of dendritic cells. J Exp Med 1998; 188:2163–2173.

157. Belz GT, Smith CM, Eichner D, et al. Conventional CD8α$^+$ dendritic cells are generally involved in priming CTL immunity to viruses. J Immunol 2004; 172: 1996–2000.

158. He Y, Zhang J, Donahue C, et al. Skin-derived dendritic cells induce potent CD8$^+$ T cell immunity in recombinant lentivector-mediated genetic immunization. Immunity 2006; 24:643–656.

159. Sharkey MS, Lizee G, Gonzales MI, et al. CD4$^+$ T-cell recognition of mutated B-RAF in melanoma patients harboring the V599E mutation. Cancer Res 2004; 64:1595–1599.

160. Yotnda P, Firat H, Garcia-Pons F, et al. Cytotoxic T cell response against the chimeric p210 BCR-ABL protein in patients with chronic myelogenous leukemia. J Clin Invest 1998; 101:2290–2296.

161. Simpson AJ, Caballero OL, Jungbluth A, et al. Cancer/testis antigens, gametogenesis and cancer. Nat Rev Cancer 2005; 5:615–625.

2

Outlining the Gap Between Preclinical Models and Clinical Situation

Daniel L. Levey

Antigenics Inc., New York, New York, U.S.A.

INTRODUCTION

This chapter discusses preclinical models of cancer immunotherapy with emphasis on autologous (i.e., personalized) approaches, and the value of these models in predicting outcomes in human disease. No model is perfect, and transplantable rodent tumor cell lines are particularly challenging tools because of their rapid rate of growth from the moment of injection. In contrast, human cancers may be latent due to slow growth over a period of many months to years before manifesting themselves. It would thus seem unlikely that a rodent tumor cell line that progresses from an inoculum to a lethal mass four weeks later can teach us anything about the human disease. Nevertheless, because models of spontaneous tumors are not amenable to autologous immunotherapy approaches comprising each tumor's unique constellation of mutated antigens, we currently must rely on established cell lines that generally become selected for rapidly dividing clones. Despite this challenging setting, the literature definitively shows that treatment of rodents with minimal tumor burden (wherein treatment begins no later than about 10 days post-tumor challenge or within a few days of surgical resection of the primary tumor) with personalized cancer vaccines improves survival to a significant degree. Such efficacy has been observed using several vaccine approaches. Treatment of longer established disease is less effective with these same approaches. Encouragingly, evidence has accumulated beyond just the anecdotal that the lives of human patients with minimal residual disease are extended with autologous immunotherapy. It is therefore apparent that immunotherapy in preclinical models tells us something about immunotherapy of human cancers. Personalized cancer immunotherapy is also amenable to combination drug treatment as a considerable body of literature demonstrates, and the value of preclinical models of such vaccine/drug cocktails is also discussed. Combination approaches are likely to be required for extending the application of cancer immunotherapy beyond early-stage disease. Drugs and biologics that slow the rate of tumor growth and/or counteract specific immune suppression will be the key components of such combination approaches.

PREDICTIVE VALUE OF PRECLINICAL MODELS

Cancer vaccines have been extensively characterized in the preclinical setting, providing a strong foundation and supporting rationale for studies in humans. Several approaches are described in this section (non-exhaustive list):

- Tumor-derived heat shock protein-peptide complexes (HSPPCs)
- Tumor cells modified to secrete cytokines
- Tumor cells modified to express costimulatory B7 molecules
- Tumor cells mixed with the adjuvant bacille Calmette–Guérin (BCG)
- Lymphoma-derived immunoglobulin (idiotype)

Two key points emerge from these studies. First, therapeutic vaccination against cancer results in benefit to the host, as measured by complete tumor rejection, prolonged stabilization of tumor growth, and/or improved survival time. The evidence for this point is extensive and based on a large variety of tumor models (described below). Second, where examined, efficacy has been observed to be greater in the minimal disease setting compared with the setting of more advanced disease. This second point echoes the case of successful early intervention against established smallpox infection: If smallpox vaccine is administered within one to four days of exposure to the disease, it may prevent or lessen the degree of illness; however, the effect of vaccination is limited if administered once disease symptoms have already started (1,2).

Transplantable tumor lines have been used in most preclinical immunotherapy studies, including chemically induced tumor lines and tumor lines of spontaneous origin. As transplantable tumors tend to become selected during passage for rapidly dividing clones that form palpable tumors within a few days after implantation in rodents, limitations on their utility arise. The most significant problem is the short lifespan of such tumor-bearing animals (typically 3–6 weeks) and thus the narrow window in which to administer the immunotherapeutic and see benefit. As amplification of an immune response takes time, the rapidly dividing tumor may outpace the development of sufficient numbers of immune effector cells. This is a major limitation of current preclinical models.

Studies showing that large numbers of tumor-specific T cells isolated from a tumor immune donor can induce tumor regression upon adoptive transfer to a tumor-bearing syngeneic recipient, highlight this kinetics problem, and offer a potential solution, although a particularly daunting one in practice (3–5).

One might consider turning to more recently developed models of spontaneous tumors in rodents where the latency period between the transforming events and the lethal tumor-bearing state is relatively long and thus provides a more realistic window for immune activation. Unfortunately, these models are not amenable to treatment with personalized vaccines that are produced from each individual host's tumor for at least two reasons. The first is practical. One must wait for a large enough primary tumor mass and/or metastases to develop such that sufficient tissue can be harvested for vaccine production. This assumes surgery can be performed on individual mice, that mice survive surgery on potentially multiple anatomical sites, that the window for immune activation after surgery and prior to death due to tumor recurrence will be wide enough, and that surgery can be performed on sufficient numbers of individual mice to run studies that stand up to statistical scrutiny. Second, the models where mice develop spontaneous tumors driven by viral oncogenes like SV40 T antigen under a tissue-specific promoter (e.g., RIP-TAg model) are complicated by the expression of the dominant viral protein in the tumor itself. This expression would likely mask or make irrelevant any immune response to individualized antigens and does not reflect the antigen profile of most tumors in humans where viral proteins are not a component of the proteome (6). This second issue may be less of a concern with other transgenic models where mammalian oncogenes are manipulated to drive transformation or where tumor suppressor genes are deleted (7,8). However, the practical reasons related to surgery on individual mice apply to these models as well. In conclusion, models of spontaneous tumor formation are really only useful for testing off-the-shelf, shared antigen vaccines.

Various approaches to immunotherapy in preclinical models are discussed below, and details of studies comparing the relative efficacy in the early-stage/minimal residual disease setting versus more advanced setting are provided in Table 1.

Tumor-Derived Heat Shock Protein-Peptide Complexes

Heat shock proteins (HSPs) are a group of proteins found in all cells in all life forms. They function as chaperones, helping proteins fold while also transporting them throughout the cell. In their chaperone function, they bind with a large repertoire of proteins and peptides. Recent studies demonstrate an essential role of HSPs (complexed with antigenic peptides) in the priming of immune response by cells undergoing necrotic death (22).

Tumor-derived complexes of HSPs and their associated peptides have been tested extensively in animal models of cancer. The published literature indicates that HSPPCs are active against established disease in nine tumor models tested,

Table 1 Examples of Preclinical Activity in Rodents Treated with Autologous Cancer Vaccines: Effect of Tumor Burden on Outcome

Cancer type	Vaccine type	Efficacy	Disease settings
Fibrosarcoma	HSPPC-96	100% complete tumor rejection (cure) in early setting vs. 0% cure in advanced disease setting (9)	Early: treatment started 5 days after tumor challenge Advanced: treatment started 9 days after tumor challenge
Lung	HSPPC-96	100% of mice alive at day 33 in vaccine group in early setting compared with 4% in control group ($P < .04$) vs. 60% survival in advanced disease (9)	Early: treatment started 5 days after surgical resection of primary tumor Advanced: treatment started 9 days after surgical resection of primary tumor
Glioma	GM-CSF–transduced tumor cells	36% prolongation of mean survival time (MST) over control treatment ($P = .0012$) in early setting vs. no difference in MST in advanced disease (10)	Early: treatment started 3 days after tumor challenge Advanced: treatment started 10 days after tumor challenge
Melanoma	GM-CSF–transduced tumor cells	40% of mice alive at day 60 (end of study) in vaccine group in early setting compared with 0% in control group ($P < .04$) vs. no difference in survival in advanced disease (11)	Early: treatment started 3 days after tumor challenge Advanced: treatment started 7 days after tumor challenge
Leukemia	GM-CSF–transduced tumor cells	100% of mice alive at day 100 (end of study) in early setting compared with 0% in control group vs. 0% alive in advanced disease (12)	Early: treatment started 1 day after tumor challenge Advanced: treatment started 7 days after tumor challenge
Mastocytoma	IL-12–transduced tumor cells	80% complete tumor rejection (cure) in early setting vs. 43% cure in moderately advanced disease setting and 14% cure in advanced disease setting (13)	Early: treatment started 6 days after tumor challenge Moderately advanced: treatment started 10 days after tumor challenge Advanced: treatment started 14 days after tumor challenge

Breast	IL-2–transduced tumor cells	100% complete tumor rejection (cure) in early setting vs. 60% cure in moderately advanced disease setting and 30% cure in advanced disease setting (14)	Early: treatment started 1 day after tumor challenge Moderately advanced: treatment started 7 days after tumor challenge Advanced: treatment started 14 days after tumor challenge
Kidney	IL-4–transduced tumor cells	70% of mice alive at day 200 (end of study) in early setting compared with 0% in control group vs. 20% alive in advanced disease (15)	Early: treatment started 6 days after tumor challenge Advanced: treatment started 9 days after tumor challenge
Mesothelioma	B7-1–transduced tumor cells	Significant reduction in rate of tumor growth in minimal disease setting vs. no effect of vaccination in bulky disease setting (16)	Minimal disease: primary tumor surgically removed prior to start of vaccination, yet still bore second tumor at distal site Bulky disease: no surgical resection and thus bore primary and secondary tumor at time of vaccination
Myeloma	TNF-α–transduced and B7-1–transduced tumor cells	87% complete tumor rejection (cure) in early setting vs. 0% cure in moderately advanced disease setting (17)	Early: treatment started 3 days after tumor challenge Moderately advanced: treatment started 7–10 days after tumor challenge
Fibrosarcoma	IFN-γ–transduced and B7-1–transduced tumor cells	83% of mice alive at day 71 (end of study) in early setting, 34% alive in moderately advanced disease setting, and 0% alive in advanced disease setting (18)	Early: treatment started 3 days after tumor challenge Moderately advanced: treatment started 10 days after tumor challenge Advanced: treatment started 17 days after tumor challenge

(Continued)

Table 1 Examples of Preclinical Activity in Rodents Treated with Autologous Cancer Vaccines: Effect of Tumor Burden on Outcome (*Continued*)

Cancer type	Vaccine type	Efficacy	Disease settings
Liver	Tumor cells mixed with BCG	33% of mice alive at end of study (>180 days) in early setting compared with 0% in control group vs. 13% alive in advanced disease (19)	Early: treatment started 10 days after tumor challenge Advanced: treatment started 20 days after tumor challenge
Liver	Tumor cells mixed with BCG	40% of mice alive at end of study (>180 days) in early setting compared with 0% in control group vs. 0% alive in advanced disease (20)	Early: treatment started 1 day after tumor challenge Advanced: treatment started 4 days after tumor challenge
Lymphoma	Adenovirus-encoding idiotype + cyclophosphamide	23% of mice alive at end of study (>60 days) in early setting compared with 0% in control group vs. 0% alive in advanced disease (21)	Early: treatment started same day as tumor challenge Advanced: treatment started 3 days after tumor challenge

Abbreviations: HSPPC-96, heat shock protein–peptide complex; GM-CSF, granulocyte macrophage colony–stimulating factor; IL-12, interleukin 12; IL-2, interleukin 2; IL-4, interleukin 4; TNF-α, tumor necrosis factor α; IFN-γ, interferon γ; BCG, bacille Calmette–Guérin.

including fibrosarcoma, leukemia, melanoma, and lung, colon, prostate, and breast cancers (9,23–28). Across these studies, HSPs have been shown to significantly slow tumor growth, elicit complete tumor regression, and/or prolong survival.

Cytokine-Secreting Tumor Cells

Tumor cells that have been modified to produce cytokines such as interleukin 2 (IL-2), IL-6, IL-12, interferon γ (IFN-γ), macrophage colony-stimulating factor (M-CSF), and granulocyte-macrophage colony-stimulating factor (GM-CSF) have been evaluated as vaccine preparations in models of established disease. Two related types of cancer cells—3LL Lewis and D122 lung cancer cells— have been widely utilized in these studies. At least 10 studies testing autologous, cytokine-producing 3LL or D122 cells in therapy have demonstrated significant benefit (29–38). Other published rodent models in which autologous, cytokine-producing tumor cells have demonstrated significant antitumor activity in therapeutic settings include models of melanoma, sarcoma, glioma, lymphoma, leukemia, squamous cell carcinoma, mastocytoma, mesothelioma, and prostate, breast, kidney, colon, bladder, and pancreatic cancers (10–15,39–51).

B7-Expressing Tumor Cells

Proper activation of the immune system requires not only presentation of antigens on the surface of antigen-presenting cells but also expression of the B7 family of costimulatory proteins. Therefore, one strategy in cancer vaccine development is the modification of tumor cells to express B7 in order to make the tumor cells more immunogenic. This vaccine strategy often includes cytokine treatment as well to further enhance immunogenicity.

In animal studies of this approach, complete regression of established tumors and/or prolongation of survival have been demonstrated in models of myeloma, hepatoma, glioma, fibrosarcoma, lymphoma, mesothelioma, mastocytoma, melanoma, and breast and colon cancers (16–18,52–58).

Tumor Cells Mixed with BCG

Another method of autologous immunotherapy involves vaccination with whole tumor cells mixed with the adjuvant BCG, which is designed to enhance immune response to vaccination. A variant of this approach is to first modify the tumor cells with a hapten, followed by mixing the cells with BCG prior to administration. The hapten binds to proteins on the tumor cell, which is believed to further increase the immunogenicity of the vaccine.

A number of studies have examined the efficacy of autologous hapten-modified or unmodified tumor cells mixed with BCG in treatment of cancer in rodents. Among the benefits observed in the studies were significant improvements in relapse-free survival and overall survival in models in which the primary tumor is surgically removed. In other models, improvement in overall survival and reduction in the metastatic disease burden in lungs were observed. Animal models included those for breast, liver, and bladder cancers (19,20,59–65).

Lymphoma-Derived Immunoglobulin (Idiotype)

Idiotype is the unique antigenic portion of the immunoglobulin produced by cancerous B cells, such as those found in lymphomas and myelomas. The idiotype protein itself or the DNA encoding the idiotype have been used as experimental autologous vaccines to generate immune response against the specific cancer from which the protein or DNA were derived.

In rodent models of established lymphoma and myeloma, a variety of idiotype vaccine approaches have demonstrated significant survival benefit. Generally, optimal efficacy has been achieved using the specific idiotype protein or encoding DNA in combination with other nonspecific immune modulators (e.g., IL-2, IL-12, GM-CSF, Flt3 ligand) or cyclophosphamide chemotherapy. In some studies, dendritic cells pulsed with the idiotype protein were used to treat mice as a form of cellular immunotherapy (21,66–69).

DO THE PRECLINICAL STUDIES PREDICT OUTCOMES IN HUMAN TRIALS?

In the clinical setting, a number of studies have tested many of the same personalized vaccine approaches described above in patients with melanoma, colon cancer, non–small cell lung cancer, and lymphoma (Table 2). Among these were two randomized, controlled trials where efficacy findings can be interpreted

Table 2 Examples of Clinical Activity in Patients Treated with Autologous Cancer Vaccines: Effect of Tumor Burden on Outcome

Treatment	Indication	Comments	Reference
HSPPC-96 (Oncophage®/ Vitespen)	Stage IV metastatic melanoma (randomized study)	M1a patients in the vaccine arm survived longer than those in the PC arm (626 vs. 383 days, $P = .177$). Survival was comparable in both arms for M1b patients (297 vs. 320 days, $P = .478$), and longer in the PC arm for M1c patients (299 vs. 226 days, $P = .015$). Impact of number of doses was examined using landmark analyses to correct potential biases. Patients who received >10 doses of vaccine survived longer than those who received PC (478 vs. 377 days, $P = .072$).	70

(Continued)

Table 2 Examples of Clinical Activity in Patients Treated with Autologous Cancer Vaccines: Effect of Tumor Burden on Outcome (*Continued*)

Treatment	Indication	Comments	Reference
Cytokine (GM-CSF)–secreting tumor cells	Stage IV metastatic melanoma (single-arm study)	28 patients treated with planned three vaccinations. 6/9 patients with non-assessable disease (e.g., NED) at time of first vaccination experienced prolonged survival (>5 yr). No patients with assessable disease were 5-yr survivors.	71
Hapten-modified irradiated tumor cells + BCG	Stage III melanoma rendered NED by surgery (single-arm study)	214 patients treated with 6–12 vaccinations. Overall survival was 61.9% in patients with a palpable lymph node mass only vs. 43.2% in patients with palpable mass plus 1–2 microscopically positive nodes and 21.4% in patients with palpable mass plus three or more microscopically positive nodes.	72
Irradiated tumor cells + BCG	Stage II and III colon cancer rendered NED by surgery (randomized study)	254 patients randomized: 128 treated with up to four vaccinations; 126 observation control. Recurrence free survival was significantly improved in vaccinated stage II patients vs. stage II control patients. No such benefit observed in stage III patients.	73
Irradiated tumor cells + BCG	Stage I, II, and III non-small cell lung cancer (single-arm study)	18 patients were treated with three vaccinations. With median follow-up of 17 mo (range 5–29 mo) since first vaccination, 8/10 stage I patients were NED and 9/10 were alive while 7/7 stage II and III patients had relapsed with 3/7 alive. The 18th patient had stage IV disease and relapsed/alive.	74
Idiotype + adjuvant	Stage II, III, and IV B cell NHL (single-arm study)	41 patients treated with five vaccinations after first undergoing standard chemotherapy. 15/21 patients who were in complete clinical remission after chemotherapy remained tumor-free with 4.6 yr median follow-up from start of vaccination. 16/20 patients with tumor present after chemotherapy experienced disease progression after vaccination.	75

Abbreviations: HSPPC, heat shock protein–peptide complex; PC, physician's choice; NED, no evidence of disease; OS, overall survival; PD, progressive disease; CR, complete response; PR, partial response.

with some confidence. Caution is more appropriate when drawing conclusions from the remaining nonrandomized studies that enrolled, in most cases, small numbers of patients. What is encouraging, however, is the consistency of the trend across multiple indications toward benefit in the setting of minimal disease versus bulky disease.

RECENT TRENDS IN PRECLINICAL MODELING

The correlation between the successful preclinical application of personalized cancer immunotherapy in early-stage disease and growing evidence for clinical activity using these same approaches in early-stage cancer patients bodes well for a field that has struggled for many decades to emerge from a morass. As cancer diagnostics continue to improve, one might predict an increase in the number of patients whose cancer is detected earlier and who would thus be amenable to personalized cancer immunotherapy. Evidence from recent clinical studies suggests that many of these patients will experience a significant improvement in recurrence free and overall survival by vaccination in the postsurgical adjuvant setting. Yet is there a role for personalized immunotherapy in patients whose disease is *not* detected early and who thus face a poorer prognosis? The preclinical models suggest that active immunotherapy alone will be insufficient to provide a meaningful impact on lifespan in this setting. Instead, as is often the case in cancer care, personalized immunotherapy will likely be used in combination with traditional cancer drugs (chemotherapeutic agents) and with other immunomodulatory agents several of which are still in experimental testing in humans. The remainder of this chapter describes some of these trends with an emphasis on preclinical experiments. In some cases, off-the-shelf (nonpersonalized) cancer vaccines that have been tested in combination with other agents are discussed. There is every reason to believe that personalized vaccines will also be useful in these combination settings.

The challenge posed by the narrow window between tumor challenge and death in preclinical models is even more pronounced in combination therapy where at least two agents are intended to be administered, in many cases in a staggered manner. In most combination studies, therefore, rodents with relatively early-stage disease have been tested. This setting, then, does not in fact perfectly mimic the advanced-stage setting in humans where drug combinations are likely to be needed. Starting treatment with a cytotoxic agent when the tumor burden in rodents is minimal may not mimic the extent of antigen release in the form of apoptosis and secondary necrosis that is expected to occur in humans with bulky disease administered the same drug. Nevertheless, the preclinical models at least provide an opportunity to determine whether the combination agent of interest is antagonistic, additive, or synergistic with immunotherapy. Assuming an additive or synergistic effect is noted, the rationale for testing in advanced-stage cancer patients will be strengthened.

Chemotherapy Plus Active Immunotherapy

Chemotherapeutic agents have been tested with cancer vaccines and have demonstrated synergy in several models. For instance, docetaxel administered two days prior to each of the three vaccinations of GM-CSF-secreting B16 melanoma cells results in 50% long-term survival of B16 tumor–bearing mice compared to 10% survival with either agent alone (76). While docetaxel was shown to induce neutropenia and lymphopenia, the expansion and survival of antigen-specific T cells (examined in OT-1 TCR transgenic mice using OVA-transfected B16 cells) was not impaired. In another study using *neu* transgenic mice, three different chemotherapeutic drugs (cyclophosphamide, doxorubicin, and paclitaxel) were tested in combination with a HER-2/neu expressing tumor vaccine and showed enhanced activity in a therapeutic setting (77). Whether drug was administered before or after vaccination affected the outcome and the optimal order of administration was found to vary from one drug to the next.

Some recent clinical studies provide yet another somewhat surprising perspective on how active immunotherapy might synergize with chemotherapy. With the caveat associated with retrospective analysis, 25 patients with glioblastoma multiforme were vaccinated with DCs loaded with autologous tumor HLA-eluted peptides or tumor lysate (78). Thirteen of these patients went on to receive subsequent chemotherapy. An additional 13 nonvaccinated patients analyzed in this study also received chemotherapy. Of the vaccine plus chemotherapy-treated patients, 42% were two-year survivors while only 8% of patients treated with chemotherapy alone or vaccine alone survived this long. It is hypothesized that infiltrating CD8+ T cells may upregulate markers on the tumor (e.g., Fas), which render cells more susceptible to chemotherapeutic drugs that kill targets via induction of apoptosis.

In another study, a striking response rate of 62% among 21 extensive-stage small cell lung cancer patients treated with second-line chemotherapy was observed after vaccination with DCs transduced with full-length p53 (79). Thirteen of the 21 patients were platinum-resistant and 61.5% of these were responders. In a third study of patients with various metastatic cancers treated with a DNA vaccine encoding a common tumor antigen, five of six immune responders who received subsequent salvage therapy experienced unexpected clinical benefit (80). Among those benefiting from the salvage therapy were four patients with progressive disease after vaccination. Among eight patients who did not demonstrate immunity to vaccination and who survived to receive additional therapy, only one derived clinical benefit.

Clearly, determining the optimal mode of administration represents a challenge to clinical applications of vaccine/chemotherapy combinations, as the best regimen may only be understood through an extensive matrix of combination testing in clinical trials. Furthermore, as discussed by Lake and Robinson, delivery of more antigen by vaccination may not be necessary in cases where the chemotherapeutic agent alone results in sufficient antigen release via tumor cell apoptosis and secondary necrosis (81). In these situations, amplification of endogenous responses to cross-presented antigen using antibodies against, e.g., CD40, may be sufficient to realize clinical benefit (82).

Nonspecific Immune Modulation Plus Active Immunotherapy

Another trend emerging in the practice of active immunotherapy with personalized (and nonpersonalized) cancer vaccines is their use in combination with other nonspecific immunomodulatory agents. Again, these combination approaches are likely to be necessary in any setting more advanced than minimal residual disease (83). Moreover, if the nonspecific agents prove to be well tolerated with minimal toxicity, there may be incentive to employ them even in the setting of minimal disease burden to further decrease the likelihood of disease recurrence. The nonspecific agents include antibodies against CTLA-4 that are designed to prevent effector T cell downregulation and a large number of agents that address the problem of immune suppression in tumor-bearing hosts. With emphases on pre-clinical testing, these various agents are discussed in turn below.

Striking synergy between anti-CTLA-4 antibody and autologous GM-CSF-secreting B16 melanoma and SM1 breast tumor vaccines against established disease in mice has been observed, and the antibody has also been tested in combination with an off-the-shelf GM-CSF-secreting prostate cancer vaccine, with promising results in preclinical studies (84–86). In a preliminary study in human cancer patients previously treated with either autologous or off-the-shelf cancer vaccines who went on to receive infusion with anti-CTLA-4 antibody, only those patients who received the autologous vaccine demonstrated signals of clinical activity (87). Many additional clinical trials are underway testing anti-CTLA-4 antibody either as monotherapy or in combination with off-the-shelf peptide vaccines, GM-CSF, and off-the-shelf whole cell vaccines (88,89 and http://www.clinicaltrials.gov/). Unfortunately, there are no clinical trials currently underway testing anti-CTLA-4 antibody with personalized cancer vaccines despite the suggestion that autologous vaccines may be a particularly potent partner for this antibody. Will the dose of antibody required vary depending on what vaccine type is employed? This later question is of interest given the autoimmune-like toxicities associated with the antibody (90).

In the last 10 to 15 years, the issue of specific immune suppression in tumor-bearing hosts has moved from a concept with few tangible toe holds from which to direct therapeutic intervention to remarkable progress in identifying molecular structures and cell types that are ripe for targeting in preclinical and clinical settings. One can envision that just as different chemotherapeutics have been combined in the clinic based on unique mechanisms of action, multiple agents each working to address distinct pathways of immune suppression will be utilized in combination. A nonexhaustive list of agents, their biological targets and evidence, where available, for utility in combination with cancer vaccines are presented in Table 3. Two agents that address the problem posed by accumulation of regulatory T cells (Tregs) are discussed in some detail.

Table 3 Selected Mechanisms of Immune Suppression in Tumor-Bearing Hosts and Intervening Strategies

Form of immunosuppression	Therapeutic agent	Mechanism of action	Preclinical evidence for synergy with cancer vaccines (selected examples)	Reference
Accumulation of $CD4^+CD25^+$ regulatory T cells (Tregs) expressing GITR and FoxP3 → reduces effector T cell function	Cyclophosphamide	Induces apoptosis in Tregs and/or downregulation of GITR and FoxP3 gene expression	See text	91–94
	Ontak	Binds to high-affinity IL-2 receptor expressed on Tregs; death by intracellular accumulation of toxin	See text	95–100
Accumulation of immature myeloid cells (ImCs) → loss of TCR ξ chain; block production of IFN-γ by T cells	All-*trans*-retinoic acid (ATRA)	Induces differentiation of ImCs; restores "normal" myeloid dendritic cell/plasmacytoid dendritic cell ratio	Mice with 4–5 mm C3 or 3–5 mm Meth A fibrosarcomas treated with tumor-specific peptide in CFA or DCs transduced with p53, respectively + implanted ATRA pellet: tumor size reduced 3–5-fold *vs.* control	101–103
Elevated levels of indoleamine 2,3-dioxygenase (IDO) in APCs and tumor cells that degrades tryptophan → effector T cell anergy/apoptosis	1-methyl-tryptophan (1MT)	Competitive inhibitor of IDO, thus preventing tryptophan catabolism	No published studies testing MT1 in combination with cancer vaccines.	104

(Continued)

Table 3 Selected Mechanisms of Immune Suppression in Tumor-Bearing Hosts and Intervening Strategies (*Continued*)

Form of immunosuppression	Therapeutic agent	Mechanism of action	Preclinical evidence for synergy with cancer vaccines (selected examples)	Reference
B cell production of CCL4 → recruits $CD4^+CD25^+$ Tregs; B cell–DC interaction → promotes IL-4, IL-10 production	Rituxan or other B cell–depleting antibodies	Deplete B cells to eliminate their deleterious effects on anti-tumor immunity	Tumor growth slower and metastases reduced in Met129 breast tumor–bearing mice partially depleted of B cells with anti-IgG/IgM sera; prolonged survival in transgenic B cell–deficient mice bearing B16 tumors vaccinated with adenovirus encoding TRP-2 compared with tumor–bearing w.t. control mice	105–111
B7-H1 expression on tumors → interacts with PD-1 on effector T cells → inhibits T cell proliferation and cytokine secretion	Blockade with anti-PD-1 or anti-B7-H1 antibodies; complete binding with soluble PD-1	Prevent effector T cell downregulation upon infiltration into tumor bed	83% long–term survival (80 days) in B16 tumor bearing mice injected with autologous HSP70 based vaccine in combination with gene encoding soluble PD-1 vs. 0% survival in controls	112–116

Cyclophosphamide has been a mainstay of cancer therapy and is typically used in combination with other chemotherapeutic drugs. In these settings, cyclophosphamide is administered at a dose that optimally causes cross-linking of DNA of rapidly dividing malignant cells. Cyclophosphamide has also been shown to have a role in immune modulation as elucidated by Robert North and others (91). It was shown that at certain doses, typically lower than those required for direct antitumor activity, cyclophosphamide selectively inhibits the activity of suppressor T cells, or what are now more commonly referred to as Tregs. This observation has been exploited in several models where the drug is given prior to administration of cancer vaccines. The premise behind this regimen is that elimination of Tregs will relieve a brake on endogenous effector T cells and/or on novel T cell specificities primed by vaccination. Berd and colleagues have combined low-dose cyclophosphamide treatment with a hapten-modified autologous melanoma vaccine strategy for many years in clinical trials (Table 2), and a pivotal study testing this approach in melanoma patients is underway (http://www.clinicaltrials.gov/). Preclinical experiments in a murine breast cancer model, also using low-dose cyclophosphamide in combination with hapten-modified autologous tumor cells, have added to the validity behind this combination approach (92). The mechanism by which cyclophosphamide inhibits the activity of Tregs in murine models is suggested to involve reduction in cell number (via apoptosis) and downregulation of GITR and FoxP3 gene expression (93,94). Given the favorable safety profile generally associated with low-dose cyclophosphamide administration and the increased understanding of its specific effect on Tregs that would allow its effectiveness to be monitored, one could envision the drug's incorporation into any number of active immunotherapy trials with the goal of reducing the deleterious effect of suppressor T cells in tumor-bearing hosts.

Ontak (denileukin diftitox) is an IL-2-diptheria toxin fusion protein that binds to the high-affinity IL-2 receptor and causes cell death. Ontak is FDA approved for treatment of cutaneous T cell lymphoma where it acts directly on malignant cells. Given that immunosuppressive T cells also express the high-affinity IL-2 receptor, recent and intensive preclinical and clinical efforts has ensued to determine whether Ontak might be useful in treatment of a number of malignancies (95–100). One of these studies tested Ontak in renal cell carcinoma patients in combination with an autologous vaccine consisting of DCs transfected with tumor-derived RNA (100). Associated with the elimination of Tregs in mice and humans treated with Ontak is enhanced levels of immunity to subsequent vaccination with various immunogens, providing a strong rationale for its ongoing investigation in immunotherapy of cancer when combined with patient-specific or off-the-shelf cancer vaccines.

CONCLUSIONS

A wealth of data suggests that preclinical models of cancer, despite their limitations, have been reasonably effective in predicting the minimal disease setting where active specific immunotherapy is most likely to be of benefit to cancer patients. Although not the focus of this chapter, it is also clear that this very setting is the most challenging in which to perform clinical trials. Patients with early-stage disease live longer and, depending on the indication, will likely have all visible disease completely resected. This leaves time to recurrence and overall survival as the only reasonable markers of efficacy of subsequently administered adjuvant immunotherapy. Although these are "gold standard" endpoints, trials in this setting can easily extend beyond five years depending on the indication. Despite this challenge, glimmers of success of autologous cancer vaccine strategies have emerged and have grown more convincing during the last decade. Looking forward, preclinical trends suggest that the tools exist to incrementally extend active, personalized immunotherapy to later stages of disease. As is often the practice in oncology, individual drugs that each address a distinct disease pathway (e.g., anti-angiogenesis, immune suppression) will likely be used in combination with therapeutic vaccines in this later stage. As this setting is relatively more difficult to model due to the rapid rate of growth of rodent tumors, it may prove necessary to look for evidence of additive or synergistic effects in small clinical trials without the full complement of preclinical testing that is more feasible in early stage disease.

REFERENCES

1. Massoudi MS, Barker L, Schwartz B. Effectiveness of postexposure vaccination for the prevention of smallpox: results of a delphi analysis. J Infect Dis 2003; 188(7):973–976.
2. Mortimer PP. Can postexposure vaccination against smallpox succeed? Clin Infect Dis 2003; 36(5):622–629.
3. Berendt MJ, North RJ. T-cell-mediated suppression of anti-tumor immunity. An explanation for progressive growth of an immunogenic tumor. J Exp Med 1980; 151(1):69–80.
4. Turk MJ, Guevara-Patino JA, Rizzuto GA, et al. Concomitant tumor immunity to a poorly immunogenic melanoma is prevented by regulatory T cells. J Exp Med 2004; 200(6):771–782.
5. Muranski P, Boni A, Wrzesinski C, et al. Increased intensity lymphodepletion and adoptive immunotherapy: how far can we go? Nat Clin Pract Oncol 2006; 3(12):668–681.
6. Gingrich JR, Barrios RJ, Morton RA, et al. Metastatic prostate cancer in a transgenic mouse. Cancer Res 1996; 56(18):4096–4102.
7. Green JE, Hudson T. The promise of genetically engineered mice for cancer prevention studies. Nat Rev Cancer 2005; 5(3):184–198.
8. Levy F, Colombetti S. Promises and limitations of murine models in the development of anticancer T-cell vaccines. Int Rev Immunol 2006; 25(5–6):269–295.
9. Kovalchin JT, Murthy AS, Horattas MC, et al. Determinants of efficacy of immunotherapy with tumor-derived heat shock protein gp96. Cancer Immun 2001; 1:7–16.
10. Herrlinger U, Kramm CM, Johnston KM, et al. Vaccination for experimental gliomas using GM-CSF-transduced glioma cells. Cancer Gene Ther 1997; 4(6): 345–352.

11. Qin H, Chatterjee SK. Cancer gene therapy using tumor cells infected with recombinant vaccinia virus expressing GM-CSF. Hum Gene Ther 1996; 7(15):1853–1860.

12. Hsieh CL, Pang VF, Chen DS, et al. Regression of established mouse leukemia by GM-CSF-transduced tumor vaccine: implications for cytotoxic T lymphocyte responses and tumor burdens. Hum Gene Ther 1997; 8(16):1843–1854.

13. Fallarino F, Ashikari A, Boon T, et al. Antigen-specific regression of established tumors induced by active immunization with irradiated IL-12- but not B7-1-transfected tumor cells. Int Immunol 1997; 9(9):1259–1269.

14. Cavallo F, Di Pierro F, Giovarelli M, et al. Protective and curative potential of vaccination with interleukin-2-gene-transfected cells from a spontaneous mouse mammary adenocarcinoma. Cancer Res 1993; 53(21):5067–5070.

15. Golumbek PT, Lazenby AJ, Levitsky HI, et al. Treatment of established renal cancer by tumor cells engineered to secrete interleukin-4. Science 1991; 254(5032): 713–716.

16. Mukherjee S, Nelson D, Loh S, et al. The immune anti-tumor effects of GM-CSF and B7-1 gene transfection are enhanced by surgical debulking of tumor. Cancer Gene Ther 2001; 8(8):580–588.

17. Xiang J, Chen Y, Moyana T. Combinational immunotherapy for established tumors with engineered tumor vaccines and adenovirus-mediated gene transfer. Cancer Gene Ther 2000; 7(7):1023–1033.

18. Yang S, Vervaert CE, Seigler HF, et al. Tumor cells cotransduced with B7.1 and gamma-IFN induce effective rejection of established parental tumor. Gene Ther 1999; 6(2):253–262.

19. Key ME, Brandhorst JS, Hanna MG Jr. Synergistic effects of active specific immunotherapy and chemotherapy in guinea pigs with disseminated cancer. J Immunol 1983; 130(6):2987–2992.

20. Hanna MG Jr., Peters LC. Specific immunotherapy of established visceral micrometastases by BCG-tumor cell vaccine alone or as an adjunct to surgery. Cancer 1978; 42(6):2613–2625.

21. Timmerman JM, Caspar CB, Lambert SL, et al. Idiotype-encoding recombinant adenoviruses provide protective immunity against murine B-cell lymphomas. Blood 2001; 97(5):1370–1377.

22. Binder RJ, Srivastava PK. Peptides chaperoned by heat-shock proteins are a necessary and sufficient source of antigen in the cross-priming of CD8+ T cells. Nat Immunol 2005; 6(6):593–599.

23. Tamura Y, Peng P, Liu K, et al. Immunotherapy of tumors with autologous tumor-derived heat shock protein preparations. Science 1997; 278(5335):117–120.

24. Janetzki S, Blachere NE, Srivastava PK. Generation of tumor-specific cytotoxic T lymphocytes and memory T cells by immunization with tumor-derived heat shock protein gp96. J Immunother 1998; 21(4):269–276.

25. Sato K, Torimoto Y, Tamura Y, et al. Immunotherapy using heat-shock protein preparations of leukemia cells after syngeneic bone marrow transplantation in mice. Blood 2001; 98(6):1852–1857.

26. Yedavelli SP, Guo L, Daou ME, et al. Preventive and therapeutic effect of tumor derived heat shock protein, gp96, in an experimental prostate cancer model. Int J Mol Med 1999; 4(3):243–248.

27. Di Paolo NC, Tuve S, Ni S, et al. Effect of adenovirus-mediated heat shock protein expression and oncolysis in combination with low-dose cyclophosphamide treatment on antitumor immune responses. Cancer Res 2006; 66(2):960–969.

28. Liu S, Wang H, Yang Z, et al. Enhancement of cancer radiation therapy by use of adenovirus-mediated secretable glucose-regulated protein 94/gp96 expression. Cancer Res 2005; 65(20):9126–9131.

29. Popovic D, El-Shami KM, Vadai E, et al. Antimetastatic vaccination against Lewis lung carcinoma with autologous tumor cells modified to express murine interleukin 12. Clin Exp Metastasis 1998; 16(7):623–632.

30. el-Shami KM, Tzehoval E, Vadai E, et al. Induction of antitumor immunity with modified autologous cells expressing membrane-bound murine cytokines. J Interferon Cytokine Res 1999; 19(12):1391–1401.

31. Porgador A, Bannerji R, Watanabe Y, et al. Antimetastatic vaccination of tumor-bearing mice with two types of IFN-gamma gene-inserted tumor cells. J Immunol 1993; 150(4):1458–1470.

32. Porgador A, Gansbacher B, Bannerji R, et al. Anti-metastatic vaccination of tumor-bearing mice with IL-2-gene-inserted tumor cells. Int J Cancer 1993; 53(3):471–477.

33. Porgador A, Tzehoval E, Katz A, et al. Interleukin 6 gene transfection into Lewis lung carcinoma tumor cells suppresses the malignant phenotype and confers immunotherapeutic competence against parental metastatic cells. Cancer Res 1992; 52(13):3679–3686.

34. Clary BM, Coveney EC, Blazer DGIIIrd, et al. Active immunization with tumor cells transduced by a novel AAV plasmid-based gene delivery system. J Immunother 1997; 20(1):26–37.

35. Sumimoto H, Tani K, Nakazaki Y, et al. Superiority of interleukin-12-transduced murine lung cancer cells to GM-CSF or B7-1 (CD80) transfectants for therapeutic antitumor immunity in syngeneic immunocompetent mice. Cancer Gene Ther 1998; 5(1):29–37.

36. Heike Y, Takahashi M, Ohira T, et al. Genetic immunotherapy by intrapleural, intraperitoneal and subcutaneous injection of IL-2 gene-modified Lewis lung carcinoma cells. Int J Cancer 1997; 73(6):844–849.

37. Morita T, Ikeda K, Douzono M, et al. Tumor vaccination with macrophage colony-stimulating factor-producing Lewis lung carcinoma in mice. Blood 1996; 88(3):955–961.

38. Lee CT, Wu S, Ciernik IF, et al. Genetic immunotherapy of established tumors with adenovirus-murine granulocyte-macrophage colony-stimulating factor. Hum Gene Ther 1997; 8(2):187–193.

39. Dranoff G, Jaffee E, Lazenby A, et al. Vaccination with irradiated tumor cells engineered to secrete murine granulocyte-macrophage colony-stimulating factor stimulates potent, specific, and long-lasting anti-tumor immunity. Proc Natl Acad Sci USA 1993; 90(8):3539–3543.

40. Abdel-Wahab Z, Dar MM, Hester D, et al. Effect of irradiation on cytokine production, MHC antigen expression, and vaccine potential of interleukin-2 and interferon-gamma gene-modified melanoma cells. Cell Immunol 1996; 171(2):246–254.

41. Sampson JH, Archer GE, Ashley DM, et al. Subcutaneous vaccination with irradiated, cytokine-producing tumor cells stimulates CD8+ cell-mediated immunity against tumors located in the "immunologically privileged" central nervous system. Proc Natl Acad Sci USA 1996; 93(19):10399–10404.

42. Schmidt W, Maass G, Buschle M, et al. Generation of effective cancer vaccines genetically engineered to secrete cytokines using adenovirus-enhanced transferrinfection (AVET). Gene 1997; 190(1):211–216.

43. Kircheis R, Kupcu Z, Wallner G, et al. Cytokine gene-modified tumor cells for prophylactic and therapeutic vaccination: IL-2, IFN-gamma, or combination IL-2 + IFN-gamma. Cytokines Cell Mol Ther 1998; 4(2):95–103.

44. Vlk V, Rossner P, Indrova M, et al. Interleukin-2 gene therapy of surgical minimal residual tumour disease. Int J Cancer 1998; 76(1):115–119.

45. Levitsky HI, Montgomery J, Ahmadzadeh M, et al. Immunization with granulocyte-macrophage colony-stimulating factor-transduced, but not B7-1-transduced, lymphoma cells primes idiotype-specific T cells and generates potent systemic antitumor immunity. J Immunol 1996; 156(10):3858–3865.

46. Myers JN, Mank-Seymour A, Zitvogel L, et al. Interleukin-12 gene therapy prevents establishment of SCC VII squamous cell carcinomas, inhibits tumor growth, and elicits long-term antitumor immunity in syngeneic C3H mice. Laryngoscope 1998; 108(2):261–268.

47. Vieweg J, Rosenthal FM, Bannerji R, et al. Immunotherapy of prostate cancer in the Dunning rat model: use of cytokine gene modified tumor vaccines. Cancer Res 1994; 54(7):1760–1765.

48. Coveney E, Clary B, Iacobucci M, et al. Active immunotherapy with transiently transfected cytokine-secreting tumor cells inhibits breast cancer metastases in tumor-bearing animals. Surgery 1996; 120(2):265–272.

49. Nagai E, Ogawa T, Kielian T, et al. Irradiated tumor cells adenovirally engineered to secrete granulocyte/macrophage-colony-stimulating factor establish antitumor immunity and eliminate pre-existing tumors in syngeneic mice. Cancer Immunol Immunother 1998; 47(2):72–80.

50. Saito S, Bannerji R, Gansbacher B, et al. Immunotherapy of bladder cancer with cytokine gene-modified tumor vaccines. Cancer Res 1994; 54(13):3516–3520.

51. Clary BM, Coveney EC, Blazer DG IIIrd, et al. Active immunotherapy of pancreatic cancer with tumor cells genetically engineered to secrete multiple cytokines. Surgery 1996; 120(2):174–181.

52. Liu Y, Wang H, Zhao J, et al. Enhancement of immunogenicity of tumor cells by cotransfection with genes encoding antisense insulin-like growth factor-1 and B7.1 molecules. Cancer Gene Ther 2000; 7(3):456–465.

53. Joki T, Kikuchi T, Akasaki Y, et al. Induction of effective antitumor immunity in a mouse brain tumor model using B7-1 (CD80) and intercellular adhesive molecule 1 (ICAM-1; CD54) transfection and recombinant interleukin 12. Int J Cancer 1999; 82(5):714–720.

54. Yi P, Yu H, Ma W, et al. Preparation of murine B7.1-glycosylphosphatidylinositol and transmembrane-anchored staphylococcal enterotoxin. A dual-anchored tumor cell vaccine and its antitumor effect. Cancer 2005; 103(7):1519–1528.

55. Douin-Echinard V, Bornes S, Rochaix P, et al. The expression of CD70 and CD80 by gene-modified tumor cells induces an antitumor response depending on the MHC status. Cancer Gene Ther 2000; 7(12):1543–1556.

56. Gaken JA, Hollingsworth SJ, Hirst WJ, et al. Irradiated NC adenocarcinoma cells transduced with both B7.1 and interleukin-2 induce CD4+-mediated rejection of established tumors. Hum Gene Ther 1997; 8(4):477–488.

57. Martin-Fontecha A, Cavallo F, Bellone M, et al. Heterogeneous effects of B7-1 and B7-2 in the induction of both protective and therapeutic anti-tumor immunity against different mouse tumors. Eur J Immunol 1996; 26(8):1851–1859.

58. La Motte RN, Rubin MA, Barr E, et al. Therapeutic effectiveness of the immunity elicited by P815 tumor cells engineered to express the B7-2 costimulatory molecule. Cancer Immunol Immunother 1996; 42(3):161–169.

59. Sojka DK, Felnerova D, Mokyr MB. Anti-metastatic activity of hapten-modified autologous tumor cell vaccine in an animal tumor model. Cancer Immunol Immunother 2002; 51(4):200–208.

60. Hoover HC Jr., Peters LC, Brandhorst JS, et al. Therapy of spontaneous metastases with an autologous tumor vaccine in a guinea pig model. J Surg Res 1981; 30(4): 409–415.

61. Peters LC, Brandhorst JS, Hanna MG Jr. Preparation of immunotherapeutic autologous tumor cell vaccines from solid tumors. Cancer Res 1979; 39(4):1353–1360.

62. Peters LC, Hanna MG Jr. Active specific immunotherapy of established micrometastasis: effect of cryopreservation procedures on tumor cell immunogenicity in guinea pigs. J Natl Cancer Inst 1980; 64(6):1521–1525.

63. Hanna M, Brandhorst J, Peters L. Active-specific immunotherapy of residual micrometastases: An evaluation of sources, doses and ratios of BCG with tumor cells. Cancer Immunol Immunother 1979; 7:165–173.

64. Hanna MG Jr., Peters LC. Immunotherapy of established micrometastases with Bacillus Calmette-Guerin tumor cell vaccine. Cancer Res 1978; 38(1):204–209.

65. Tzai TS, Huben RP, Zaleskis G, et al. Effect of perioperative chemoimmunotherapy with cyclophosphamide and autologous tumor vaccine in murine MBT-2 bladder cancer. J Urol 1994; 151(6):1680–1686.

66. Chen HW, Lee YP, Chung YF, et al. Inducing long-term survival with lasting anti-tumor immunity in treating B cell lymphoma by a combined dendritic cell-based and hydrodynamic plasmid-encoding IL-12 gene therapy. Int Immunol 2003; 15(3): 427–435.

67. Campbell MJ, Esserman L, Levy R. Immunotherapy of established murine B cell lymphoma. Combination of idiotype immunization and cyclophosphamide. J Immunol 1988; 141(9):3227–3233.

68. Zeis M, Zunkel T, Steinmann J, et al. Enhanced antitumoral effectiveness of idiotype vaccination induced by the administration of Flt3 ligand combined with interleukin 2 against a murine myeloma. Br J Haematol 2002; 117(1):93–102.

69. Stritzke J, Zunkel T, Steinmann J, et al. Therapeutic effects of idiotype vaccination can be enhanced by the combination of granulocyte-macrophage colony-stimulating factor and interleukin 2 in a myeloma model. Br J Haematol 2003; 120(1):27–35.

70. Richards J, Testori A, Whitman E, et al. Autologous tumor-derived HSPPC-96 vs. physician's choice (PC) in a randomized phase III trial in stage IV melanoma. J Clin Oncol, 2006 ASCO Annual Meeting Proceedings Part I. Vol 24, No. 18S (June 20 Suppl), 2006:8002.

71. Luiten RM, Kueter EW, Mooi W, et al. Immunogenicity, including vitiligo, and feasibility of vaccination with autologous GM-CSF-transduced tumor cells in metastatic melanoma patients. J Clin Oncol 2005; 23(35):8978–8991.

72. Berd D, Sato T, Maguire HC Jr., et al. Immunopharmacologic analysis of an autologous, hapten-modified human melanoma vaccine. J Clin Oncol 2004; 22(3): 403–415.

73. Vermorken JB, Claessen AM, van Tinteren H, et al. Active specific immunotherapy for stage II and stage III human colon cancer: a randomised trial. Lancet 1999; 353(9150): 345–350.

74. Schulof RS, Mai D, Nelson MA, et al. Active specific immunotherapy with an autologous tumor cell vaccine in patients with resected non-small cell lung cancer. Mol Biother 1988; 1(1):30–36.

75. Hsu FJ, Caspar CB, Czerwinski D, et al. Tumor-specific idiotype vaccines in the treatment of patients with B-cell lymphoma: long-term results of a clinical trial. Blood 1997; 89(9):3129–3135.

76. Prell RA, Gearin L, Simmons A, et al. The anti-tumor efficacy of a GM-CSF-secreting tumor cell vaccine is not inhibited by docetaxel administration. Cancer Immunol Immunother 2006; 55(10):1285–1293.

77. Machiels JP, Reilly RT, Emens LA, et al. Cyclophosphamide, doxorubicin, and paclitaxel enhance the antitumor immune response of granulocyte/macrophage-colony stimulating factor-secreting whole-cell vaccines in HER-2/neu tolerized mice. Cancer Res 2001; 61(9):3689–3697.

78. Wheeler CJ, Das A, Liu G, et al. Clinical responsiveness of glioblastoma multiforme to chemotherapy after vaccination. Clin Cancer Res 2004; 10(16):5316–5326.

79. Antonia SJ, Mirza N, Fricke I, et al. Combination of p53 cancer vaccine with chemotherapy in patients with extensive stage small cell lung cancer. Clin Cancer Res 2006; 12(3 Pt. 1):878–887.

80. Gribben JG, Ryan DP, Boyajian R, et al. Unexpected association between induction of immunity to the universal tumor antigen CYP1B1 and response to next therapy. Clin Cancer Res 2005; 11(12):4430–4436.

81. Lake RA, Robinson BW. Immunotherapy and chemotherapy: a practical partnership. Nat Rev Cancer 2005; 5(5):397–405.

82. Nowak AK, Robinson BW, Lake RA. Synergy between chemotherapy and immunotherapy in the treatment of established murine solid tumors. Cancer Res 2003; 63(15):4490–4496.

83. Lizee G, Radvanyi LG, Overwijk WW, et al. Improving antitumor immune responses by circumventing immunoregulatory cells and mechanisms. Clin Cancer Res 2006; 12(16):4794–4803.

84. van Elsas A, Hurwitz AA, Allison JP. Combination immunotherapy of B16 melanoma using anti-cytotoxic T lymphocyte-associated antigen 4 (CTLA-4) and granulocyte/macrophage colony-stimulating factor (GM-CSF)-producing vaccines induces rejection of subcutaneous and metastatic tumors accompanied by autoimmune depigmentation. J Exp Med 1999; 190(3):355–366.

85. Hurwitz AA, Yu TF, Leach DR, et al. CTLA-4 blockade synergizes with tumor-derived granulocyte-macrophage colony-stimulating factor for treatment of an experimental mammary carcinoma. Proc Natl Acad Sci USA 1998; 95(17): 10067–10071.

86. Hurwitz AA, Foster BA, Kwon ED, et al. Combination immunotherapy of primary prostate cancer in a transgenic mouse model using CTLA-4 blockade. Cancer Res 2000; 60(9):2444–2448.

87. Hodi FS, Mihm MC, Soiffer RJ, et al. Biologic activity of cytotoxic T lymphocyte-associated antigen 4 antibody blockade in previously vaccinated metastatic melanoma and ovarian carcinoma patients. Proc Natl Acad Sci USA 2003; 100(8):4712–4717.

88. Gerritsen W, Van Den Eertwegh AJ, De Gruijl TD, et al. A dose-escalation trial of GM-CSF-gene transduced allogeneic prostate cancer cellular immunotherapy in combination with fully human anti-CTL4 antibody (MDX-010, ipiluminab) in patients with metastatic hormone-refractory prostate cancer (MHRPC). Proceedings, ASCO Annual Meeting, June 1–5, 2007, Chicago (abst 262).

89. Gerritsen WR, van den Eertwegh AJ, de Gruijl TD, et al. Biochemical and immunologic correlates of clinical response in a combination trial of the GM-CSF-gene transduced allogeneic prostate cancer immunotherapy and ipilimumab in patients with metastatic hormone-refractory prostate cancer (mHRPC). J Clin Oncol, 2007 ASCO Annual Meeting Proceedings Part I. Vol 25, No. 18S (June 20 Suppl), 2007:5120.

90. Peggs KS, Quezada SA, Korman AJ, et al. Principles and use of anti-CTLA4 antibody in human cancer immunotherapy. Curr Opin Immunol 2006; 18(2):206–213.

91. North RJ. Cyclophosphamide-facilitated adoptive immunotherapy of an established tumor depends on elimination of tumor-induced suppressor T cells. J Exp Med 1982; 155(4):1063–1074.

92. Sojka DK, Felnerova D, Mokyr MB. Anti-metastatic activity of hapten-modified autologous tumor cell vaccine in an animal tumor model. Cancer Immunol Immunother 2002; 51(4):200–208.

93. Lutsiak ME, Semnani RT, De Pascalis R, et al. Inhibition of CD4(+)25+ T regulatory cell function implicated in enhanced immune response by low-dose cyclophosphamide. Blood 2005; 105(7):2862–2868.

94. Ghiringhelli F, Larmonier N, Schmitt E, et al. CD4+CD25+ regulatory T cells suppress tumor immunity but are sensitive to cyclophosphamide which allows immunotherapy of established tumors to be curative. Eur J Immunol 2004; 34(2): 336–344.

95. Mahnke K, Schonfeld K, Fondel S, et al. Depletion of CD4+CD25+ human regulatory T cells in vivo: kinetics of Treg depletion and alterations in immune functions in vivo and in vitro. Int J Cancer 2007; 120(12):2723–2733.

96. Litzinger MT, Fernando R, Curiel TJ, et al. The IL-2 immunotoxin denileukin diftitox reduces regulatory T cells and enhances vaccine-mediated T-cell immunity. Blood 2007 Jul 6; [Epub ahead of print].

97. Knutson KL, Dang Y, Lu H, et al. IL-2 immunotoxin therapy modulates tumor-associated regulatory T cells and leads to lasting immune-mediated rejection of breast cancers in neu-transgenic mice. J Immunol 2006; 177(1):84–91.

98. Attia P, Maker AV, Haworth LR, et al. Inability of a fusion protein of IL-2 and diphtheria toxin (Denileukin Diftitox, DAB389IL-2, ONTAK) to eliminate regulatory T lymphocytes in patients with melanoma. J Immunother 2005; 28(6):582–592.

99. Barnett B, Kryczek I, Cheng P, et al. Regulatory T cells in ovarian cancer: biology and therapeutic potential. Am J Reprod Immunol 2005; 54(6):369–377.

100. Dannull J, Su Z, Rizzieri D, et al. Enhancement of vaccine-mediated antitumor immunity in cancer patients after depletion of regulatory T cells. J Clin Invest 2005; 115(12):3623–3633.

101. Mirza N, Fishman M, Fricke I, et al. All-*trans*-retinoic acid improves differentiation of myeloid cells and immune response in cancer patients. Cancer Res 2006; 66(18): 9299–9307.

102. Kusmartsev S, Cheng F, Yu B, et al. All-*trans*-retinoic acid eliminates immature myeloid cells from tumor-bearing mice and improves the effect of vaccination. Cancer Res 2003; 63(15):4441–4449.
103. Kusmartsev S, Gabrilovich DI. Role of immature myeloid cells in mechanisms of immune evasion in cancer. Cancer Immunol Immunother 2006; 55(3):237–245.
104. Munn DH, Mellor AL. Indoleamine 2,3-dioxygenase and tumor-induced tolerance. J Clin Invest 2007; 117(5):1147–1154.
105. Barbera-Guillem E, Nelson MB, Barr B, et al. B lymphocyte pathology in human colorectal cancer. Experimental and clinical therapeutic effects of partial B cell depletion. Cancer Immunol Immunother 2000; 48(10):541–549.
106. Perricone MA, Smith KA, Claussen KA, et al. Enhanced efficacy of melanoma vaccines in the absence of B lymphocytes. J Immunother 2004; 27(4):273–281.
107. Inoue S, Leitner WW, Golding B, et al. Inhibitory effects of B cells on antitumor immunity. Cancer Res 2006; 66(15):7741–7747.
108. Shah S, Divekar AA, Hilchey SP, et al. Increased rejection of primary tumors in mice lacking B cells: inhibition of anti-tumor CTL and TH1 cytokine responses by B cells. Int J Cancer 2005; 117(4):574–586.
109. Bystry RS, Aluvihare V, Welch KA, et al. B cells and professional APCs recruit regulatory T cells via CCL4. Nat Immunol 2001; 2(12):1126–1132.
110. Moulin V, Andris F, Thielemans K, et al. B lymphocytes regulate dendritic cell (DC) function in vivo: increased interleukin 12 production by DCs from B cell-deficient mice results in T helper cell type 1 deviation. J Exp Med 2000; 192(4):475–482.
111. Qin Z, Richter G, Schuler T, et al. B cells inhibit induction of T cell-dependent tumor immunity. Nat Med 1998; 4(5):627–630.
112. Blank C, Mackensen A. Contribution of the PD-L1/PD-1 pathway to T-cell exhaustion: an update on implications for chronic infections and tumor evasion. Cancer Immunol Immunother 2007; 56(5):739–745.
113. Geng H, Zhang GM, Xiao H, et al. HSP70 vaccine in combination with gene therapy with plasmid DNA encoding sPD-1 overcomes immune resistance and suppresses the progression of pulmonary metastatic melanoma. Int J Cancer 2006; 118(11):2657–2664.
114. Hirano F, Kaneko K, Tamura H, et al. Blockade of B7-H1 and PD-1 by monoclonal antibodies potentiates cancer therapeutic immunity. Cancer Res 2005; 65(3): 1089–1096.
115. Li N, Qin H, Li X, et al. Potent systemic antitumor immunity induced by vaccination with chemotactic-prostate tumor associated antigen gene-modified tumor cell and blockade of B7-H1. J Clin Immunol 2007; 27(1):117–130.
116. Iwai Y, Terawaki S, Honjo T. PD-1 blockade inhibits hematogenous spread of poorly immunogenic tumor cells by enhanced recruitment of effector T cells. Int Immunol 2005; 17(2):133–144.

3

Therapeutic and Prophylactic Cancer Vaccines: Emerging Perspectives from Allogeneic and Infectious Disease Vaccines

Roopa Srinivasan

Agni Consulting Services, San Marcos, California, U.S.A.

INTRODUCTION

Cancer remains a major cause of death worldwide despite multiple approaches to therapy and prevention. Nonsurgical methods of treatment include chemotherapy and/or radiotherapy that target rapidly dividing cells. Of the more recently developed treatment modalities for cancer are biological therapies such as hormonal and antibody therapeutics, and vaccines. The past two decades have seen the science of tumor immunology evolve into a distinct discipline forming the basis of cancer vaccines. Of particular relevance to the development of tumor vaccines has been the presence of immunity to tumor antigens. This is of significance, given that tumor antigens arise from self-tissue. However, the challenge of breaking through host immune tolerance to effectively mount a robust antitumor response still remains.

The immune system has evolved to combat parasites, bacteria, and viruses based on recognition of foreign antigens on these pathogens. Consequently, vaccines have been effective in the induction of protective immunity to infectious disease agents. Gardasil™ (Merck & Co., Inc., New Jersey, U.S.A.), the first cancer vaccine approved by the FDA, is a prophylactic vaccine against cervical cancer in young women (1). The vaccine is a quadrivalent virus–like particle (VLP) vaccine and offers protection by generating neutralizing antibodies against the human papillomavirus (HPV). This vaccine does not protect women who are already infected with the papilloma virus and who may consequently develop cervical cancer.

While traditionally the immune system has evolved to protect the host from invading pathogens, it is also believed to be triggered when it perceives a "danger" signal by the host's self-tissue (2). In cancer, such signals may be associated with the existence of tumor immunity as seen with clinical examples of spontaneous regressions in melanoma, gastrointestinal, lung, and breast cancers (3). In addition, histopathology of tumor sections has revealed infiltrating lymphocytes around the tumor bed, and recent studies indicate that ovarian cancer patients with such infiltrates in tumors have an improved prognosis compared with similarly staged patients without lymphocytic infiltrates (4). Therefore, the immune repertoire may contain autoreactive immune cells capable of rejecting tumors, when activated appropriately. However, in spite of clear animal model data demonstrating the potential therapeutic benefit of cancer vaccines, with the exception of those for viral-mediated cancers, therapeutic tumor vaccines have had only limited success in humans. More recent studies are looking at enhancing tumor-specific responses using immune modulators in an attempt to translate them to effective tumor protection.

Different types of cancer vaccines have induced tumor immunity and a correlative antitumor response in syngeneic mouse tumor models, leading to their efficacy testing in human. Most noteworthy examples of therapeutic cancer vaccines that are in various stages of development are plasmid or viral-vector DNA, dendritic cells (DCs) pulsed with peptide or RNA, allogeneic whole tumor cells, allogeneic tumor-cell lysate, cytokine-transduced tumor cells, heat shock proteins, and autologous T-cell therapy (5,6). Among the prophylactic vaccines, the one that was recently approved is Gardasil™ for the prevention of cervical cancer; precancerous genital lesions; and genital warts due to HPV) types 6, 11, 16, and 18 in young women (1).

Allogeneic tumor vaccines as potential form of a therapeutic vaccine were tested in large randomized phase 3 trials. The two allogeneic tumor-cell vaccines that were tested in phase 3 trials for melanoma were Melacine® (Corixa Corporation Washington, U.S.A./GlaxoSmithKline, England, UK) and Canvaxin™ (CancerVax Corporation, California, U.S.A./Micromet, Inc., Maryland, U.S.A.). Both vaccines had showed efficacy in the early stages of clinical development. However, pivotal trials did not indicate a clinical benefit and the trials were discontinued. Phase 3 trials with GVAX® (Cell Genesys, California, U.S.A.) are ongoing for the treatment of prostate cancer. In this chapter, we will discuss the potential that some of the allogeneic tumor vaccines have offered and the reasons for their failure in becoming a successful therapeutic agent. We will also examine the possible criteria that contributed to the success of Gardasil™ and consider some of these ideas in the development of therapeutic cancer vaccines.

ALLOGENEIC VACCINES

There is growing evidence that a variety of cancers can be clinically treated by vaccines. This was seen in two randomized phase 3 studies where an autologous tumor-cell-vaccine approach as an adjuvant for the treatment of colorectal and renal cancers provided clinical benefit (7,8). Several vaccine strategies (DC/peptide or RNA, protein or DNA) have employed a single-antigen approach in which either an overexpressed or uniquely expressed tumor antigen or epitope that is identified on tumor tissue is targeted. The limitation of this approach lies in both the chosen antigen as well as the major histocompatibility complex type of the patient (in the case of peptide immunization). Polyvalent tumor vaccines that are allogeneic or autologous should, at least in theory, overcome these limitations.

Tumor cells as polyvalent vaccines have been attractive as they are the richest source of antigens. With a wide array of potential tumor antigens (some or possibly most of them unknown), they could potentially activate and amplify every facet of the immune system for both cellular and humoral antitumor responses. These cell lines can be manipulated in vitro, such as addition of cytokine genes to enhance potential antitumor effect (9). In addition (as with whole tumor-cell vaccines), professional antigen-presenting cells (APCs) such as DCs may phagocytize apoptotic tumor cells from the vaccine and effectively cross-prime T cells with a host of immunogenic epitopes (10).

Added to its therapeutic appeal is the idea that allogeneic vaccines share a manufacturing advantage. Allogeneic cell lines for use as whole cells, lysates, or genetic manipulations can be initially difficult to establish in vitro and they require antigenic consistency and proof of stability. However, once established, this approach provides unlimited material for vaccination by overcoming the requirement for tumor tissue and/or leukapheresis from the patient (as for some autologous vaccines) and consequently the delay in preparation of vaccine. They can be consistently manufactured in large lots that can be used to treat multiple patients and be fully tested before release. Whole tumor cells, lysates, and genetically modified tumors have been tried as allogeneic vaccines in clinical trials.

Allogeneic Whole Tumor Cells

Some of the earliest attempts at inducing an antitumor response were in melanoma, where intact allogeneic cell lines were used as a vaccine (11). Canvaxin™ is a whole, multicell polyvalent vaccine consisting of a mixture of three sublethally irradiated allogeneic melanoma lines that are of different HLA haplotypes expressing various known tumor antigens (12). Canvaxin™ has the potential benefit of viable but nonreplicating cells so that they may continue to express and present antigen. Tumor-cell profiling by flow cytometry indicated the expression of gangliosides, tyrosinase, TRP-1/gp75, Melan-A, and gp100. The assurance that irradiation of the final product is effective and that cells have been rendered replication-incompetent is of critical importance for allogeneic tumor whole-cell vaccines. This was achieved at irradiation doses at which the cell could not replicate while maintaining antigenic integrity.

Canvaxin™ was extensively tested in phase 1 and 2 clinical trials with the results indicating a statistically significant increase in median and five-year survival of stage III and IV surgically resected patients with melanoma when compared with matched historical controls (13,14). The promising clinical benefit was correlated with vaccine-induced immune responses (11,15–18). Early phase 2 nonrandomized clinical trial results indicated a strong cellular delayed type hypersensitivity (DTH) along with high anti-TA99 IgM and anti-GD2, -GD3, -GM2, and -GM3 ganglioside IgM titers in patients with resected melanoma (19). Serum complement–dependent cytotoxicity for melanoma cell lines in vitro also increased over baseline levels when patients were administered this polyvalent vaccine (15). Canvaxin™ was tested in a postsurgical adjuvant setting in large double-blinded, randomized phase 3 trials for AJCC stage III and IV melanoma (20,21). The trials compared patients vaccinated with either Canvaxin™ or placebo, with both arms having received BCG with the first two doses. All patients were observed for overall survival (OS) and disease-free survival (DFS). In spite of encouraging immune responses to Canvaxin™ in early studies, both trials were discontinued because the independent Data and Safety Monitoring Board found that the data were unlikely to provide significant evidence of an OS benefit for these melanoma patients treated with Canvaxin™, when compared with those on the control arm (6,22,23). The control arm in these pivotal trials, which included BCG without the allogeneic cell component of the vaccine, did better than expected. The vaccinated patients in phase 1 and 2 trials were compared to matched historical controls that did not receive BCG.

Autologous tumor vaccines, with BCG as a component, have been shown to be effective in randomized trials for stage II and III colon carcinoma (7,24,25). While the importance of randomized phase 2 trials is becoming increasingly recognized and implemented, it is perhaps crucial when immune adjuvants form a component of the vaccine regimen.

Allogeneic Tumor-Cell Lysate

These vaccines are conceptually similar to whole-cell vaccines, except that protein and other cellular components from the lysate serve as the immunogens. Melacine® is a mechanically disrupted cell lysate from 20×10^6 tumor-cell equivalents of two allogeneic melanoma lines given with a proprietary immunological adjuvant DETOX® (Corixa Corporation, Washington, U.S.A./ GlaxoSmithKline, England, UK) (26). Several known potential antigens such as those from the gangliosides, tyrosinase, and MAGE families as well as Melan A, gp100, and HMW-MAA were expressed by these cell lines.

A phase 1 trial in melanoma patients indicated a clinical response in 5 out of 17 patients (27). Clinical response was correlated with the presence of cytotoxic T lymphocytes (CTLs) and antibodies and a DTH response against melanoma antigens. Phase 1 and 2 trials conducted on AJCC stage IV patients indicated that 6% of the patients showed an objective response. The vaccine also indicated a well-tolerated safety profile. This modest antitumor activity in stage IV melanoma patients led to the licensure of Melacine® in Canada for use in advanced disease (28).

The promise of this vaccine in an adjuvant setting was tested in a large phase 3 trial with surgically resected lesions of intermediate thickness in node negative melanoma patients (29,30). The premise of this trial was that these stage II patients would have a low tumor burden (T3N0M0) and less tumor-induced immune suppression providing a longer time for immune response to work against tumor. The trial compared patients vaccinated with 40 doses of Melacine® given over the first two years with those that were observed for recurrence-free survival (RFS) and OS. On the basis of a similar study with fewer patients, Mitchell and his colleagues had reported a clinical benefit in those patients who expressed HLA types A2, A28, B44, B45, and C3, with the strongest benefit in those patients expressing HLA A2 and/or C3 (31). Both RFS and OS in the pivotal trial were significantly increased in HLA A2/C3 melanoma patients (26). However, no significant improvement in RFS or OS was observed in the test population as a whole (which included patients expressing other HLA types as well). Prospective randomized trials would be needed to confirm the clinical benefit of this type of vaccine in defined HLA A2/C3 subsets in the adjuvant setting before the approach can be considered as providing therapeutic benefit.

Cytokine-Modified Tumor Vaccine

Several cytokines such as IFN-α, IFN-γ, IL-12, and IL-2 have been used to enhance an antitumor CD8$^+$ response (32–35), of which one of the most effective cytokines used as an immune adjuvant is GM-CSF (36). GM-CSF is a powerful immune adjuvant, and attracts and activates DCs at a site of vaccination (37). Transducing polyvalent tumor cells with GM-CSF has the advantage of recruiting DCs to the vaccine where it encounters a multitude of potential tumor antigens to provide a wide-ranging and durable response. Preclinical studies in a B16 mouse–melanoma model have demonstrated that GM-CSF transduced tumor cells, in comparison to other cytokines such as IL-4 and IL-6, and induced the most potent systemic antitumor effect (36). Many subsequent studies in other murine tumor models have validated the potent systemic immunity induced by GM-CSF–transduced tumor-cell immunotherapies (38–40).

The above-mentioned approach is currently followed in clinical trials for treatment of several types of cancers (41). Tumor lines are genetically modified to secrete GM-CSF and followed by irradiation to render them incapable of proliferation. The current approach includes GM-CSF–engineered and irradiated tumor cells that are either allogeneic (patient nonspecific) or autologous (patient specific). The most mature candidate of these is GVAX®, a patient nonspecific vaccine, and is currently being studied in a phase 3 trial in patients with advanced-stage, hormone-refractory prostate cancer. This vaccine is composed of two prostate cancer cell lines: one derived from a lymph node metastasis and the other from a bone metastasis, which were genetically modified to secrete GM-CSF. Data from early trials in hormone-refractory prostate cancer indicted an enhanced survival by about seven months, on the basis of which pivotal trials are underway. Other trials using GVAX® combined with chemotherapy or immune modulators are at various stages of clinical development (9).

INFECTIOUS DISEASE VACCINES

Generation of vaccines for infectious diseases has been more successful for obvious reasons in that the antigen is foreign and the immune system can therefore mount a robust response. This vital observation by Edward Jenner in 1796 revolutionized this discipline when he inoculated people with the related cowpox virus to build immunity against the deadly smallpox virus, leading to the global eradication of the disease by 1980. Prophylactic cancer vaccines that prevent the onset of cancer have shown success in a preventative setting through neutralizing antibodies against the virus that is the causative agent for some cancers. The recently approved vaccine Gardasil™ is of prominence for cervical cancer in young women 9 to 26 years of age who are protected from the onset of infection to the HPV (1). This VLP vaccine is effective against HPV types 16 and 18, responsible for approximately 70% of cervical cancers, and against HPV types 6 and 11, which cause approximately 90% of genital warts. Cervarix™ (GlaxoSmithKline, England, UK) is another vaccine against HPV types 16 and 18 that was approved in Australia in May 2007 for use in women between 10 and 45 years of age (42). Cervarix™ is formulated with a novel proprietary adjuvant system called AS04, which is designed to enhance immune response and increase the duration of protection (43).

Vaccines for the prevention and/or treatment of other virus- and bacteria-induced cancers such as those caused by hepatitis B and hepatitis C (HBV and HCV), Epstein–Barr (EBV) viruses, and *Helicobacter pylori* are also being studied. However, in this chapter, we will restrict ourselves to information about HPV vaccines alone.

Human Papillomavirus

About 500,000 women are diagnosed with cervical cancer every year, making it the third leading cause of death in women. At least 93% of these invasive cervical cancers contain the HPV. This etiologic agent is a double-stranded DNA virus surrounded by capsid proteins, L1 and L2, and six regulatory proteins, E1, E2, E4, E5, E6, and E7. While the majority of cervical cancers and their precursor lesions contain HPV DNA (44), the expression of specifically the E6 and E7 viral proteins in precursor squamous intraepithelial lesions (SIL) leads to malignant transformation (45). HPV DNA gets integrated into the host genome in cancer cells; however, it remains in an episomal state in precancerous or noncancerous cells (46,47).

Preventative HPV vaccines were designed by expressing the capsid protein L1 in bacteria (48), yeast (49), insect (50), or mammalian systems (51,52). The expressed L1 proteins spontaneously assemble to form VLPs that do not carry the oncogenic genome. Preclinical data in rabbits and canines indicate that L1 VLPs of the cottontail rabbit papillomavirus (CRPV) and canine oral papillomavirus (COPV) could generate an antibody response that protect them from a subsequent viral challenge (53,54). Passive transfer of these antibodies from immune animals was also able to confer protection to a viral challenge in nonimmunized animals. These types of observations along with those from other investigators have led to the clinical testing and subsequent approval of the first vaccine against cervical cancer (1,55,56).

The development of antibodies to capsid VLP as a preventative vaccine is a landmark in the epidemiology of cervical cancer. However, the more challenging issue is the treatment of precursor and fully transformed cervical cancer lesions for which neutralizing antibodies are ineffective and a cell-mediated immune response is required. Though capsid proteins have also been known to generate an antigen-specific cell-mediated immunity, this does not clear those infections that are established or those that have escaped antibody surveillance (57). However, several other studies suggest that cell-mediated immune responses may control HPV-associated malignancies. Vaccinating rabbits with nonstructural viral proteins generated an immune response that induced regression of virus-induced papillomas. Although the vaccination generated antibodies, there was no correlation between antibody titers and regression, suggesting a cell-mediated mechanism of control (58). Additional evidence is seen in clinical settings when immunocompromised individuals such as transplant or HIV-positive patients have shown a higher incidence of HPV infections and associated neoplasms (59–62). Moreover, warts on patients who are on immunosuppressive therapy often disappear when the treatment is discontinued (63). In addition, infiltrating immune cells were observed in histological samples of spontaneously regressing warts (64,65).

Of the six identified regulatory proteins of HPV mentioned above, the oncogenic viral proteins E6 and E7 are required to maintain malignancy (66,67). Studies in prophylaxis and therapeutic animal models using HPV (E6/E7)-immortalized tumor cells have indicated the requirement of CD4 helper and CD8 effector T lymphocytes (68). In addition, T-cell responses against E7 are frequently seen in patients with cervical neoplasia and a persistent viral load

(69). In another study, as an indication of natural defense mechanisms against HPV-related cervical lesions, Th1 responses to in vitro peptide stimulation (of E6 and E7 oncoproteins) of lymphocytes from patients with low- to high-grade and invasive cervical cancer showed a decreasing level of IL-2 production when compared with previously infected individuals who were cytologically negative (70). The evidence of CTL responses to E6 or E7 in HPV-positive women without cervical intraepithelial neoplasia is important compared with responses in the HPV-positive women with neoplasia (71,72). These data collectively suggest that E6 and E7 may be attractive targets for a therapeutic vaccine against cervical cancer (73).

LESSONS LEARNED FROM TRADITIONAL CANCER VACCINE TRIALS AND INFECTIOUS DISEASE VACCINE MODELS

Over the past two decades, cancer vaccines as a possible treatment modality have seen much promise. While a variety of approaches in preclinical studies have induced a "cure" for mouse cancers, several of these approaches have been tried in human with limited success. The only approved therapeutic cancer vaccine, a xenogeneic DNA vaccine, was for the treatment of canine melanoma (74). However, the field has substantially matured, with information from a host of clinical trials now available to help in the understanding of major aspects of preclinical and clinical vaccine development. In contrast, infectious disease vaccines target an invading pathogen, and the success in developing this type of vaccine is inherently straightforward. Taken collectively, there are some elements from these studies that may be useful in developing therapeutic cancer vaccines regardless of whether the cancer arises from self-tissue or is induced by a pathogen.

There are several factors in the preclinical development of a vaccine that need to be considered. These include the choice of relevant target antigens, immunogenicity of the vaccine, dosing—both route of administration and timing of vaccine administration, combination of vaccine with immune modulators or other treatment modalities, and appropriate mouse models to conduct and analyze proof of concept studies. There is sufficient evidence from infectious disease and cancer immunotherapy studies that one of the appropriate types of antigens to target would be that which is imperative for a cancer cell to survive and proliferate. For example, in cervical cancer, the expression of E6 and E7 proteins of the viral genome is crucial to maintain malignancy. These are therefore expressed exclusively in cervical cancer cells and not on normal cells, making this an attractive target. Likewise, successful antibody therapies to treat several cancers have been those that target growth factor receptors, cell activation and signaling molecules, or molecules in the angiogenesis pathway. While targeting these molecules has a greater potential of autoimmune toxicity, this undesired side effect may be associated only in the face of a robust antitumor response. Clinical studies have indicated that this may be controllable or even a reversible phenomenon. Tumor load is another consideration for the success of a vaccine. Studies from mice models for cervical cancer have indicated that the antitumor therapeutic effects targeting the E7 subunit are better achieved when tumor burden is low. In addition, studies in patients have indicated that precursor lesions have been associated with a CTL response, while no CTL activity is detected when these become established cancers.

Several other methods of augmenting an immune response to tumor antigens have been studied. Examples of prime-boost strategies and use of immune modulators are among a few. Immune modulators such as Toll-like receptor (TLR) agonists to enhance antigen uptake and presentation by DCs, activation of B7 family of costimulators on DCs, and dampening of negative costimulatory molecules such as CTLA-4 on T cells have all been used separately. A probable chance of success would be achieved when using some of these modulators in combination and timing them appropriately in the vaccination schedule to obtain a robust immune response.

Among clinical studies, more thought is required into the type of patient population that should be enrolled in the study. Several clinical studies have indicted that therapeutic cancer vaccines are not effective in bulky disease, or in late- or end-stage patients. This is probably due to tumor-induced immune suppression caused by soluble factors such as TGF-β. Several studies now indicate the role of $CD4^+CD25^+$ T regulatory cells and their role in inducing tolerance. These cells depend on TGF-β for their survival and suppress T effector cytolytic function, which is considered crucial for the killing of tumor. The probability of this approach becoming a treatment option is most likely in a minimal disease setting or as an adjuvant where one would expect to find minimal tumor-induced immune suppression.

Also, an aspect of the success of pivotal trials depends on results from controlled phase 2 studies. This would eliminate an assumption that similarities exist between the two groups of patients studied at different points in time and in the face of continuous assessments and improvements on disease staging/classification and clinical/immunological monitoring. Patients may be randomized to an observation or follow-up arm, or an intent-to-treat arm of the trial, depending on the vaccine, staging of the disease, and the clinical end point. While efficacy data were often compared with historical controls, more and more phase 2 trials are now being randomized.

Of importance is the development of biomarkers and imaging techniques in aiding diagnosis and disease monitoring during treatment. In a recent study using molecular-genetic imaging techniques, the investigators showed that they could induce EBV tyrosine kinase expression within tumors by treating with Velcade®, a proteosome inhibitor, followed by radiolabeled 2'-fluoro-2'-deoxy-beta-D-5-iodouracil-arabinofuranoside (FIAU) to image and potentially kill these tumors (75). Like imaging, the use of biomarkers will be an important tool to aid monitoring in clinical trials. To name a few, markers such as prostate-specific antigen (PSA) and CA-125 are currently available to monitor the disease status of patients with prostate or ovarian carcinomas, respectively, indicating the need to identify more of these.

The development of cancer vaccines has clearly been fraught with challenges. Nevertheless, the wealth of information acquired from preclinical and clinical studies has guided us to a level where much has been learnt and new insights gained. All these lessons can potentially be exploited to chalk out various avenues to develop successful therapeutic cancer vaccines.

REFERENCES

1. Gardasil F. FDA Licenses New Vaccine for Prevention of Cervical Cancer and Other Diseases in Females Caused by Human Papillomavirus. FDA; 2006.
2. Matzinger P. The danger model: a renewed sense of self. Science 2002; 296(5566): 301–305.
3. Challis GB, Stam HJ. The spontaneous regression of cancer. A review of cases from 1900 to 1987. Acta Oncol 1990; 29(5):545–550.
4. Zhang L, Conejo-Garcia JR, Katsaros D, et al. Intratumoral T cells, recurrence, and survival in epithelial ovarian cancer. N Engl J Med 2003; 348(3):203–213.
5. Srinivasan R, Wolchok JD. Tumor antigens for cancer immunotherapy: therapeutic potential of xenogeneic DNA vaccines. J Transl Med 2004; 2(1):12.
6. Srinivasan R, Van Epps D. Specific active immunotherapy of cancer: potential and perspectives. Rev Recent Clin Trials 2006; 1:283–292.
7. Uyl-de Groot CA, Vermorken JB, Hanna MG Jr., et al. Immunotherapy with autologous tumor cell-BCG vaccine in patients with colon cancer: a prospective study of medical and economic benefits. Vaccine 2005; 23(17–18):2379–2387.
8. Jocham D, Richter A, Hoffmann L, et al. Adjuvant autologous renal tumour cell vaccine and risk of tumour progression in patients with renal-cell carcinoma after radical nephrectomy: phase III, randomised controlled trial. Lancet 2004; 363(9409): 594–599.
9. Hege KM, Jooss K, Pardoll D. GM-CSF gene-modified cancer cell immunotherapies: of mice and men. Int Rev Immunol 2006; 25(5–6):321–352.
10. Shaif-Muthana M, McIntyre C, Sisley K, et al. Dead or alive: immunogenicity of human melanoma cells when presented by dendritic cells. Cancer Res 2000; 60(22): 6441–6447.
11. Barth A, Hoon DS, Foshag LJ, et al. Polyvalent melanoma cell vaccine induces delayed-type hypersensitivity and in vitro cellular immune response. Cancer Res 1994; 54(13):3342–3345.
12. Van Epps D. Characterization of polyvalent allogeneic vaccines. Dev Biol (Basel) 2004; 116:79–90; discussion 133–143.
13. Morton DL, Hoon DS, Nizze JA, et al. Polyvalent melanoma vaccine improves survival of patients with metastatic melanoma. Ann N Y Acad Sci 1993; 690:120–134.
14. Morton DL, Foshag LJ, Hoon DS, et al. Prolongation of survival in metastatic melanoma after active specific immunotherapy with a new polyvalent melanoma vaccine. Ann Surg 1992; 216(4):463–482.
15. Hsueh EC, Famatiga E, Gupta RK, et al. Enhancement of complement-dependent cytotoxicity by polyvalent melanoma cell vaccine (CancerVax): correlation with survival. Ann Surg Oncol 1998; 5(7):595–602.

16. Hsueh EC, Essner R, Foshag LJ, et al. Active immunotherapy by reinduction with a polyvalent allogeneic cell vaccine correlates with improved survival in recurrent metastatic melanoma. Ann Surg Oncol 2002; 9(5):486–492.

17. DiFronzo LA, Gupta RK, Essner R, et al. Enhanced humoral immune response correlates with improved disease-free and overall survival in American Joint Committee on Cancer stage II melanoma patients receiving adjuvant polyvalent vaccine. J Clin Oncol 2002; 20(15):3242–3248.

18. Ravindranath MH, Hsueh EC, Verma M, et al. Serum total ganglioside level correlates with clinical course in melanoma patients after immunotherapy with therapeutic cancer vaccine. J Immunother (1997) 2003; 26(3):277–285.

19. Hsueh EC, Gupta RK, Qi K, et al. Correlation of specific immune responses with survival in melanoma patients with distant metastases receiving polyvalent melanoma cell vaccine. J Clin Oncol 1998; 16(9):2913–2920.

20. Hsueh EC, Morton DL. Antigen-based immunotherapy of melanoma: Canvaxin therapeutic polyvalent cancer vaccine. Semin Cancer Biol 2003; 13(6):401–407.

21. Morton DL, Hsueh EC, Essner R, et al. Prolonged survival of patients receiving active immunotherapy with Canvaxin therapeutic polyvalent vaccine after complete resection of melanoma metastatic to regional lymph nodes. Ann Surg 2002; 236(4): 438–448; discussion 48–49.

22. Faries MB, Morton DL. Therapeutic vaccines for melanoma: current status. BioDrugs 2005; 19(4):247–260.

23. CancerVax Corporation. Available at: http://ir.cancervax.com/phoenix.zhtml?c=147045&p=irol-newsArticle&t=Regular&id=763722&. Accessed 2005.

24. Harris JE, Ryan L, Hoover HC Jr., et al. Adjuvant active specific immunotherapy for stage II and III colon cancer with an autologous tumor cell vaccine: Eastern Cooperative Oncology Group Study E5283. J Clin Oncol 2000; 18(1):148–157.

25. Hanna MG Jr., Hoover HCJr., Vermorken JB, et al. Adjuvant active specific immunotherapy of stage II and stage III colon cancer with an autologous tumor cell vaccine: first randomized phase III trials show promise. Vaccine 2001; 19(17–19):2576–2582.

26. Sondak VK, Sosman JA. Results of clinical trials with an allogenic melanoma tumor cell lysate vaccine: Melacine. Semin Cancer Biol 2003; 13(6):409–415.

27. Mitchell MS, Kan-Mitchell J, Kempf RA, et al. Active specific immunotherapy for melanoma: phase I trial of allogeneic lysates and a novel adjuvant. Cancer Res 1988; 48(20):5883–5893.

28. Mitchell MS. Perspective on allogeneic melanoma lysates in active specific immunotherapy. Semin Oncol 1998; 25(6):623–635.

29. Sondak VK, Liu PY, Tuthill RJ, et al. Adjuvant immunotherapy of resected, intermediate-thickness, node-negative melanoma with an allogeneic tumor vaccine: overall results of a randomized trial of the Southwest Oncology Group. J Clin Oncol 2002; 20(8):2058–2066.

30. Sosman JA, Unger JM, Liu PY, et al. Adjuvant immunotherapy of resected, intermediate-thickness, node-negative melanoma with an allogeneic tumor vaccine: impact of HLA class I antigen expression on outcome. J Clin Oncol 2002; 20(8):2067–2075.

31. Mitchell MS, Harel W, Groshen S. Association of HLA phenotype with response to active specific immunotherapy of melanoma. J Clin Oncol 1992; 10(7):1158–1164.

32. Rosenberg SA, Yang JC, Schwartzentruber DJ, et al. Impact of cytokine administration on the generation of antitumor reactivity in patients with metastatic melanoma receiving a peptide vaccine. J Immunol 1999; 163(3):1690–1695.

33. Salgia R, Lynch T, Skarin A, et al. Vaccination with irradiated autologous tumor cells engineered to secrete granulocyte-macrophage colony-stimulating factor augments antitumor immunity in some patients with metastatic non-small-cell lung carcinoma. J Clin Oncol 2003; 21(4):624–630.

34. Maio M, Fonsatti E, Lamaj E, et al. Vaccination of stage IV patients with allogeneic IL-4- or IL-2-gene-transduced melanoma cells generates functional antibodies against vaccinating and autologous melanoma cells. Cancer Immunol Immunother 2002; 51(1):9–14.

35. Lee P, Wang F, Kuniyoshi J, et al. Effects of interleukin-12 on the immune response to a multipeptide vaccine for resected metastatic melanoma. J Clin Oncol 2001; 19(18):3836–3847.

36. Dranoff G, Jaffee E, Lazenby A, et al. Vaccination with irradiated tumor cells engineered to secrete murine granulocyte-macrophage colony-stimulating factor stimulates potent, specific, and long-lasting anti-tumor immunity. Proc Natl Acad Sci USA 1993; 90(8):3539–3543.

37. Bowne WB, Wolchok JD, Hawkins WG, et al. Injection of DNA encoding granulocyte-macrophage colony-stimulating factor recruits dendritic cells for immune adjuvant effects. Cytokines Cell Mol Ther 1999; 5(4):217–225.

38. Machiels JP, Reilly RT, Emens LA, et al. Cyclophosphamide, doxorubicin, and paclitaxel enhance the antitumor immune response of granulocyte/macrophage-colony stimulating factor-secreting whole-cell vaccines in HER-2/neu tolerized mice. Cancer Res 2001; 61(9):3689–3697.

39. Borrello I, Sotomayor EM, Rattis FM, et al. Sustaining the graft-versus-tumor effect through posttransplant immunization with granulocyte-macrophage colony-stimulating factor (GM-CSF)-producing tumor vaccines. Blood 2000; 95(10): 3011–3019.

40. Dunussi-Joannopoulos K, Dranoff G, Weinstein HJ, et al. Gene immunotherapy in murine acute myeloid leukemia: granulocyte-macrophage colony-stimulating factor tumor cell vaccines elicit more potent antitumor immunity compared with B7 family and other cytokine vaccines. Blood 1998; 91(1):222–230.

41. Cell Genesys, Inc. Available at: http://www.cellgenesys.com/clinical-stage.shtml. Accessed 2005.

42. Cervarix. Cervarix is approved in Australia for females 10–45 years old. GSK, 2007.

43. Harper DM, Franco EL, Wheeler CM, et al. Sustained efficacy up to 4.5 years of a bivalent L1 virus-like particle vaccine against human papillomavirus types 16 and 18: follow-up from a randomised control trial. Lancet 2006; 367(9518):1247–1255.

44. Walboomers JM, Jacobs MV, Manos MM, et al. Human papillomavirus is a necessary cause of invasive cervical cancer worldwide. J Pathol 1999; 189(1):12–19.

45. zur Hausen H. Papillomaviruses and cancer: from basic studies to clinical application. Nat Rev Cancer 2002; 2(5):342–350.

46. Cullen AP, Reid R, Campion M, et al. Analysis of the physical state of different human papillomavirus DNAs in intraepithelial and invasive cervical neoplasm. J Virol 1991; 65(2):606–612.

47. Stoler MH, Rhodes CR, Whitbeck A, et al. Human papillomavirus type 16 and 18 gene expression in cervical neoplasias. Hum Pathol 1992; 23(2):117–128.

48. Nardelli-Haefliger D, Roden RB, Benyacoub J, et al. Human papillomavirus type 16 virus-like particles expressed in attenuated *Salmonella typhimurium* elicit mucosal and systemic neutralizing antibodies in mice. Infect Immun 1997; 65(8):3328–3336.

49. Sasagawa T, Pushko P, Steers G, et al. Synthesis and assembly of virus-like particles of human papillomaviruses type 6 and type 16 in fission yeast *Schizosaccharomyces pombe.* Virology 1995; 206(1):126–135.
50. Kirnbauer R, Booy F, Cheng N, et al. Papillomavirus L1 major capsid protein self-assembles into virus-like particles that are highly immunogenic. Proc Natl Acad Sci USA 1992; 89(24):12180–12184.
51. Zhou J, Sun XY, Davies H, et al. Definition of linear antigenic regions of the HPV16 L1 capsid protein using synthetic virion-like particles. Virology 1992; 189(2):592–599.
52. Hagensee ME, Yaegashi N, Galloway DA. Self-assembly of human papillomavirus type 1 capsids by expression of the L1 protein alone or by coexpression of the L1 and L2 capsid proteins. J Virol 1993; 67(1):315–322.
53. Breitburd F, Kirnbauer R, Hubbert NL, et al. Immunization with viruslike particles from cottontail rabbit papillomavirus (CRPV) can protect against experimental CRPV infection. J Virol 1995; 69(6):3959–3963.
54. Suzich JA, Ghim SJ, Palmer-Hill FJ, et al. Systemic immunization with papillomavirus L1 protein completely prevents the development of viral mucosal papillomas. Proc Natl Acad Sci USA 1995; 92(25):11553–11557.
55. Villa LL, Costa RL, Petta CA, et al. Prophylactic quadrivalent human papillomavirus (types 6, 11, 16, and 18) L1 virus-like particle vaccine in young women: a randomised double-blind placebo-controlled multicentre phase II efficacy trial. Lancet Oncol 2005; 6(5):271–278.
56. Villa LL, Ault KA, Giuliano AR, et al. Immunologic responses following administration of a vaccine targeting human papillomavirus types 6, 11, 16, and 18. Vaccine 2006; 24(27–28):5571–5583.
57. De Bruijn ML, Greenstone HL, Vermeulen H, et al. L1-specific protection from tumor challenge elicited by HPV16 virus-like particles. Virology 1998; 250(2):371–376.
58. Selvakumar R, Borenstein LA, Lin YL, et al. Immunization with nonstructural proteins E1 and E2 of cottontail rabbit papillomavirus stimulates regression of virus-induced papillomas. J Virol 1995; 69(1):602–605.
59. Halpert R, Fruchter RG, Sedlis A, et al. Human papillomavirus and lower genital neoplasia in renal transplant patients. Obstet Gynecol 1986; 68(2):251–258.
60. Laga M, Icenogle JP, Marsella R, et al. Genital papillomavirus infection and cervical dysplasia: opportunistic complications of HIV infection. Int J Cancer 1992; 50(1):45–48.
61. Meyer T, Arndt R, Nindl I, et al. Association of human papillomavirus infections with cutaneous tumors in immunosuppressed patients. Transpl Int 2003; 16(3):146–153.
62. Petry KU, Scheffel D, Bode U, et al. Cellular immunodeficiency enhances the progression of human papillomavirus-associated cervical lesions. Int J Cancer 1994; 57(6):836–840.
63. Benton C, Shahidullah H, Hunter JAA. Human papillomavirus in the immunosuppressed. Papillomavirus Report 1992:23–26.
64. Aiba S, Rokugo M, Tagami H. Immunohistologic analysis of the phenomenon of spontaneous regression of numerous flat warts. Cancer 1986; 58(6):1246–1251.
65. Iwatsuki K, Tagami H, Takigawa M, et al. Plane warts under spontaneous regression. Immunopathologic study on cellular constituents leading to the inflammatory reaction. Arch Dermatol 1986; 122(6):655–659.
66. Munger K, Phelps WC, Bubb V, et al. The E6 and E7 genes of the human papillomavirus type 16 together are necessary and sufficient for transformation of primary human keratinocytes. J Virol 1989; 63(10):4417–4421.

67. Werness BA, Levine AJ, Howley PM. Association of human papillomavirus types 16 and 18 E6 proteins with p53. Science 1990; 248(4951):76–79.
68. Kim TY, Myoung HJ, Kim JH, et al. Both E7 and CpG-oligodeoxynucleotide are required for protective immunity against challenge with human papillomavirus 16 (E6/E7) immortalized tumor cells: involvement of CD4+ and CD8+ T cells in protection. Cancer Res 2002; 62(24):7234–7240.
69. de Gruijl TD, Bontkes HJ, Stukart MJ, et al. T cell proliferative responses against human papillomavirus type 16 E7 oncoprotein are most prominent in cervical intraepithelial neoplasia patients with a persistent viral infection. J Gen Virol 1996; 77(Pt. 9):2183–2191.
70. Tsukui T, Hildesheim A, Schiffman MH, et al. Interleukin 2 production in vitro by peripheral lymphocytes in response to human papillomavirus-derived peptides: correlation with cervical pathology. Cancer Res 1996; 56(17):3967–3974.
71. Nakagawa M, Stites DP, Farhat S, et al. Cytotoxic T lymphocyte responses to E6 and E7 proteins of human papillomavirus type 16: relationship to cervical intraepithelial neoplasia. J Infect Dis 1997; 175(4):927–931.
72. Nakagawa M, Stites DP, Patel S, et al. Persistence of human papillomavirus type 16 infection is associated with lack of cytotoxic T lymphocyte response to the E6 antigens. J Infect Dis 2000; 182(2):595–598.
73. Sin JI, Hong SH, Park YJ, et al. Antitumor therapeutic effects of e7 subunit and DNA vaccines in an animal cervical cancer model: antitumor efficacy of e7 therapeutic vaccines is dependent on tumor sizes, vaccine doses, and vaccine delivery routes. DNA Cell Biol 2006; 25(5):277–286.
74. Animal Medical Center. Canine Melanoma Vaccine Clinical Trial for USDA Licensure and Commercial Use. Animal Medical Center; 2007.
75. Fu DX, Tanhehco YC, Chen J, et al. Virus-associated tumor imaging by induction of viral gene expression. Clin Cancer Res 2007; 13(5):1453–1458.

4

Personalized Cancer Vaccines

Florentina Teofilovici and Kerry Wentworth
Antigenics Inc., Lexington, Massachusetts, U.S.A.

THERAPEUTIC CANCER VACCINES VS. TRADITIONAL CANCER TREATMENT

Traditional cancer drugs are cytotoxic agents, meaning that they kill cells. Although most chemotherapeutics preferentially affect rapidly dividing cells (i.e., cancer cells), they cannot differentiate between malignant and normal cells. The unavoidable toxicity to normal cells often results in treatment-related toxicities such as increased susceptibility to bleeding and infection, mucositis, nausea and vomiting, hair loss, etc. This nonspecific approach to cancer treatment makes it more suitable for use in disease settings in which the tumor burden is high, such as advanced or metastatic disease.

Therapeutic cancer vaccines belong to a newer class of targeted cancer therapies. Like innovative treatments such as Gleevec® (imatinib mesylate; Novartis, New Jersey, U.S.) and Herceptin® (trastuzumab; Genentech, California, U.S.), most cancer vaccines in development are designed to attack only malignant cells. By targeting tumor cells with high specificity, this new class of treatments tends to be associated with fewer toxicities compared with traditional cancer drugs.

The discovery that cancer regression can be achieved when antigens (substances capable of triggering immune response) on malignant cells are recognized by the immune system means that, theoretically, malignant cells can be eradicated without toxicity to normal, healthy tissues.

In 1908, Paul Ehrlich and Ilya Mechnikov were awarded the Nobel Prize for their hypothesis of the immune surveillance theory of cancer, which suggested that the immune system continually "removes" tumors that arise spontaneously (1). Their theories lay largely dormant until it was noticed a half century later that Kaposi's sarcoma occurred in kidney transplant recipients whose immune systems were pharmacologically suppressed to allow their transplanted organ to "take." Once immunosuppression was stopped, the tumors regressed (2–5).

At this time, Klein et al. demonstrated the phenomenon that one could immunize against tumors in the same manner as was being performed with remarkable success against polio and smallpox viruses (6,7). It was known that although tumors are of self-origin (in contrast with viruses), they are still capable of triggering an immune response. From this observation, researchers correctly predicted that tumors must express tumor-specific antigens that are responsible for triggering this response. Burnett also suggested that transplantation antigens expressed on tumor cells could stimulate the immune system, leading to the generation of "protective" immunity that prevented against tumor development (8,9). Recently, use of a new generation of mice with deficient immune systems has solidified the crucial role of the immune system in protecting against spontaneous tumors (10).

The increased risk of cancers in patients with medically induced primary or acquired immunosuppression has firmly established a role for the immune system in the control of cancer (11). The tumors observed in medically immunosuppressed organ transplant patients are similar to cancers seen in individuals infected with human immunodeficiency virus (HIV). HIV patients have a 10,000-fold increased risk of developing blood cancers as well as a significantly higher incidence of other cancers (11,12). However, similar to immunosuppression-induced cancers in transplant recipients, cancers often regress when an HIV patient's immune system is restored using highly active antiretroviral therapy (13–15). The clear demonstration of a relationship between the immune system and cancer has led to the development of many therapeutic cancer vaccines.

PERSONALIZED CANCER VACCINES

Despite the varied approaches employed by the many therapeutic cancer vaccines in development, they all share one fundamental goal: to program a patient's immune system to attack the patient's cancer. Some vaccines utilize antigens (any substance capable of stimulating an immune response) that are known to be associated with certain types of tumors. In recent years, there was an increased interest on so-called unique antigens that are products of random mutations arising in the course of tumor cells' uncontrolled cell divisions. This led researchers' interest and work on personalized (autologous) cancer vaccines that use the patients' own tumor cells to generate immune response specific to the patients' own cancers. Pramod Srivastava, Professor of Immunology and Director of the University of Connecticut Cancer Center explains, "A cancer cell can host millions of mutant peptides. Each time a cell divides, it probably has about somewhere between 6 and 60 mutations" (16).

The personalized vaccines have the opportunity to present to the host immune system the entire repertoire of the mutated peptides (antigens capable of triggering immune system response) resulted from the degradation of encoded proteins. The vaccines prepared from patient's own tumor have the advantage of possibly being more immunogenic, exposing the host immune system to a perceived "foreign" large number of muted peptides including those antigens that researchers have not yet recognized.

Another approach in personalized cancer vaccines is the dendritic cell–based therapy. Patient's dendritic cells (DC) are stimulated ex vivo through exposure to tumor-cell lysate, fusion with tumor cells, infected by virus containing a gene or exposure to purified peptides. A single or a few peptides from cancer-specific antigens can be used to pulse the patient's own DC. Given back to the patient, DC will present the tumor antigens to the T cells in the effector arm of the immune system (17).

In contrast to personalized vaccines using patient's own tumor to derive a large repertoire of antigens that DC load in vivo, DC vaccines are using patient's own blood to process autologous DC that are loaded in the laboratory with allogeneic tumor antigens expressed by the majority of tumors in a given type of cancer or on a variety of cancers.

Whether they are based on cancer cells, purified proteins, or live immune cells, most therapeutic cancer vaccines generally aim to activate the branch of the immune system that can directly target and specifically kill cancer cells.

Therapeutic cancer vaccines are based on the principle that, given the right conditions, the human immune system is capable of generating an effective antitumor immune response.

CLINICAL DATA IN PERSONALIZED CANCER VACCINES THAT REACHED PHASE 3 CLINICAL TRIALS

One of the shared and clear advantages to cancer vaccines is the excellent safety profile, which makes their use in the adjuvant or earlier-stage disease setting more suitable than more conventional treatments such as chemotherapy. Choudhury et al. note that "collectively the data indicate that vaccine therapy is safe, and no significant autoimmune reactions are observed even on long-term follow-up" (18). Such a safety profile would indicate the potential for a high quality of life index, which is a unique feature when measured against the adverse effects associated with traditional cancer treatments.

Despite a general consensus that cancer vaccines appear to be safe and well tolerated, it is more difficult to draw conclusions regarding their efficacy. To date, there have only been approximately 25 randomized phase 2 or 3 trials conducted with cancer vaccines. However, there are several examples that indicate treatment activity is present in subsets of cancer patients and, as predicted by the preclinical studies, this activity is typically seen in earlier stages of disease. The following sections have the description of the autologous cancer vaccines that reached the phase 3 development and the related clinical trial results (summary of the vaccine information is provided in Table 1).

Table 1 Personalized Cancer Vaccines: Characteristics

Vaccine	Class of vaccine	Composition	Target tumor/ indication	Lead phase of development
OncoVAX®	Polyvalent	Autologous-irradiated tumor cells mixed with adjuvant BCG	Colon cancer, adjuvant setting	Phase 3
Oncophage®	Polyvalent	Autologous tumor-derived heat shock protein-peptide complex gp96	Renal cell carcinoma, adjuvant setting	Phase 3
Provenge®	Dendritic cells	Autologous dendritic cells and a fusion protein composed of PAP and GM-CSF	Prostate cancer, metastatic HRPC	Phase 3
Favld®	Antigen specific	Autologous recombinant anti-idiotype protein conjugated to KLH, administered with GM-CSF	Follicular B-cell non-Hodgkin's lymphoma following treatment with Rituxan®	Phase 3
MyVax®	Antigen specific	Autologous recombinant anti-idiotype protein conjugated to KLH, administered with GM-CSF	Untreated follicular non-Hodgkin's lymphoma	Phase 3

Abbreviations: BCG, bacille Calmette–Guérin; PAP, prostatic acid phosphatase; GM-CSF, granulocyte-macrophage colony-stimulating factor; KLH, keyhole limpet hemocyanin; HRPC, hormone-refractory prostate cancer.

OncoVAX® (Intracel; Frederick, MD, U.S.)

OncoVAX is an autologous vaccine prepared individually from each patient's tumor cells. After surgical resection of the tumor, cells from the tumor are irradiated and then mixed with the adjuvant bacille Calmette–Guérin (BCG, an attenuated strain of bacteria that can boost immune response to a vaccine). It is designed to stimulate a specific immune response against each patient's own cancer.

OncoVAX was evaluated in the adjuvant setting (in conjunction with another treatment—in this case, surgery) in a phase 3 clinical trial involving patients with stage II and III colon cancer. In the study, patients were randomized to receive either OncoVAX or observation after surgical resection of the primary tumor. The study found that with a 5.8-year median follow-up, there was a statistically significant benefit associated with vaccine for both recurrence-free survival and overall survival (OS) in stage II (earlier-stage) patients ($n = 157$) but not in stage III (advanced-stage) patients ($n = 84$). In the trial, OncoVAX was associated with a significant improvement in five-year recurrence-free survival (79% vs. 62% for vaccine and control groups, respectively; $P = 0.009$). OS was also significantly improved in stage II patients receiving vaccine (82.5%) compared with comparable patients in the control arm (72.7%; $P = 0.010$) (19). A phase 3 confirmatory trial in stage II colon cancer is planned.

Oncophage® (Vitespen; Antigenics, Lexington, MA, U.S.)

Oncophage is an autologous vaccine that consists of complexes of heat shock proteins (HSPs) and their associated peptides derived from patients' own tumor cells. These complexes (HSPPCs) comprise a sort of antigenic "fingerprint" that is unique to each patient's cancer. The vaccine is designed to stimulate a specific immune response against cancer cells bearing this fingerprint.

Oncophage was evaluated in a phase 3 study, which randomized 728 patients with nonmetastatic renal cell carcinoma (RCC; kidney cancer) at high risk for recurrence to receive either nephrectomy alone (observation arm) or nephrectomy plus Oncophage vaccination. Subgroup analyses demonstrated that in 361 patients (60% of randomized eligible patients) with earlier-stage disease and it increased risk of recurrence [stage I (high histological grade), stage II (high-grade), or stage III T1, T2, and T3a (low-grade)] treatment with Oncophage resulted in prolonged time to recurrence ($P < 0.01$; HR $= 0.550$) (20).

ATL (Reniale®; LipoNova AG, Hannover, Germany)

Reniale is an autologous cancer vaccine based on lysates from patient's tumor cells. The cells are purified and after a few hours of incubation with gamma interferon they go through a devitalization process.

Liponova completed a phase 3 trial of Reniale, involving 558 patients with nonmetastatic RCC. Although the majority of clinical research indicates greater benefit of cancer vaccines among patients with earlier-stage disease, a subset analysis of the phase 3 trial found a significant reduction in tumor progression for patients with T3 tumors but not those with T2 tumors (21). Five-year progression-free survival (PFS) was 81.3% for patients with T2 tumors who received vaccine ($n = 119$) versus 74.6% for similar patients in the control arm ($n = 145$; $P = 0.216$). For patients with T3 tumors, five-year PFS was 67.5% for those in the vaccine arm ($n = 58$) compared with 49.7% for those in the control arm ($n = 57$; $P = 0.039$). Liponova provided an updated report with additional OS data (22). This secondary intent-to-treat (ITT) analysis was performed on 477 patients (233 patients in the treatment group and 244 patients in the control group). PFS remained in favor of the Reniale group ($P = 0.0476$, log-rank test), with no statistically significant OS difference between both groups. In the per protocol group, there remained 134 patients in the Reniale group and 218 patients in the control group where both PFS and OS were statistically significant in favor of the Reniale group ($P = 0.024$, log-rank test, for PFS; and $P = 0.0356$, log-rank test, for OS, respectively).

Provenge® (Sipuleucel-T; Dendreon, Seattle, WA, U.S.)

Provenge consists of autologous (patient-derived) DC that have been cultured with a "delivery cassette" that contains a version of the prostate cancer–associated antigen prostatic acid phosphatase (PAP) (found in about 95% of prostate cancers) and the cytokine granulocyte-macrophage colony-stimulating factor (GM-CSF). It is designed to activate specialized immune cells called T cells to recognize and destroy cells bearing the PAP antigen. In contrast to personalized vaccines using patient's own tumor to derive a large repertoire of antigens, Provenge uses a generic antigen common in prostate carcinoma. A phase 3 trial of Provenge involving 127 patients with asymptomatic, androgen-independent, metastatic prostate cancer (study D9901) missed the primary end point of time to progression. However, the final three-year follow-up data showed a median survival benefit of 21%, or 4.5 months, and a threefold improvement in survival at 36 months compared with placebo, regardless of Gleason score ($P = 0.010$; HR = 1.7) (23).

A second phase 3 trial (study D9902A), involving 98 men with asymptomatic, metastatic, androgen-independent prostate cancer, corroborated findings from the first trial: Patients who received vaccine had a 19.0-month median survival time compared with 15.7 months for patients who received placebo, representing a 21% improvement ($P = 0.331$; HR = 1.3). Integrated analysis of data from both trials showed a statistically significant survival benefit among the overall ITT population of 225 patients: Patients who received Provenge had a median survival of 23.2 months compared with 18.9 months for patients who received placebo ($P = 0.011$; HR = 1.5) (24). A third, pivotal phase 3 trial (study D9902B) is ongoing to evaluate Provenge as a treatment for advanced prostate cancer.

CANCER VACCINES: ONGOING PHASE 3 STUDIES

FavId® (Favrille; San Diego, CA, U.S.)

FavId is an autologous active cancer immunotherapy in which recombinant patient-specific idiotype protein isolated from tumor biopsy is conjugated to keyhole limpet hemocyanin (KLH) and administered in combination with the immunostimulatory factor GM-CSF. FavId is currently undergoing a phase 3 clinical study to determine its ability to extend time to progression (TTP) in patients with follicular B-cell non-Hodgkin's lymphoma following treatment with Rituxan®. The primary end point is disease-free survival at three years. At the time of the prospectively planned interim analysis conducted on 233 out of 349 randomized patients who had been followed for 12 months or more (25), there was no significant difference between FavId-treated and control groups in a secondary end point of response improvement; final data are expected at the end of 2007 (26).

MyVax® (GTOP; Genitope Corporation, Fremont, CA, U.S.)

MyVax personalized immunotherapy is an autologous active cancer immunotherapy consisting of recombinant patient-specific idiotype that is conjugated to KLH, an immunogenic carrier protein, and administered along with GM-CSF adjuvant. Results from a phase 2 study showed that 9 of the 21 patients in the study remained progression-free in their last clinical follow-up at 56 to 78 months following chemotherapy. A pivotal phase 3 study to measure PFS in patients with follicular non-Hodgkin's lymphoma is underway and scheduled to be completed by December 2007 (27).

Stimuvax® (Biomira; Edmonton, AB, Canada/Merck KGaA, Darmstadt, Germany)

Stimuvax, a non-patient-specific vaccine, consists of a synthetic peptide derived from the tumor-associated antigen MUC-1 encapsulated in a liposome (a phospholipid shell intended to facilitate and improve treatment delivery). It is designed to neutralize the immunosuppressive effect of MUC-1 to better enable the immune system to target the cancer.

A phase 2, randomized, open-label trial evaluated Stimuvax in patients with stage IIIB or IV non-small cell lung cancer (NSCLC) whose disease was stable or had responded to treatment following completion of first-line standard chemotherapy, with or without radiation treatment. Final analysis of the trial, which involved 171 patients, showed a survival advantage associated with vaccination for patients with stage IIIB disease (earlier-stage disease and therefore associated with better prognosis; $n = 65$) but not for patients with stage IV disease (advanced-stage disease, worse prognosis; $n = 106$) (28,29). In the study, median survival was 30.6 months for stage IIIB patients who received vaccine compared with 13.3 months for stage IIIB patients in the control arm (best supportive care based on current standard clinical practice, which includes palliative radiation therapy and/or second-line chemotherapy). A 1300-patient phase 3 trial has recently launched in patients with stage IIIA or IIIB locoregional NSCLC (30).

GSK 1572932A (GlaxoSmithKline; Philadelphia, PA, U.S.)

This cancer immunotherapeutic non-patient-specific vaccine consists of a purified recombinant MAGE-A3 protein combined with GSK's proprietary adjuvant system. The agent is designed to trigger an immune response against tumor cells expressing MAGE-A3, a tumor-specific antigen expressed on a variety of cancers including NSCLC and melanoma.

GlaxoSmithKline has initiated a phase 3, randomized, double-blind placebo-controlled trial of GSK 1572932A as an adjuvant therapy in patients with stage IB, II, or IIIA resectable NSCLC whose tumors express the MAGE-A# antigen. The study will enroll approximately 2270 patients and the primary end point is disease-free survival. GSK 1572932A is used in combination with VaxImmune and QS-21 Stimulon adjuvants (30).

THE CONVENTIONAL DRUG DEVELOPMENT MODEL AND DIFFICULTIES APPLYING REGULATORY PROCESS TO CANCER VACCINE DEVELOPMENT

The conventional development model for new treatments consists of preclinical and clinical research phases. Preclinical research entails laboratory studies to investigate the basic properties of a drug as well as studies in animals to evaluate the safety and efficacy of a treatment in animal "models" of human diseases.

Clinical research is the investigation of an experimental treatment in humans. Clinical trials are designed to answer specific questions about new therapies or new ways of using known treatments. They are used to determine whether a new drug or treatment is both safe and effective, and are only conducted if the preclinical studies have yielded promising results. Before a treatment is approved for marketing, clinical research is typically divided into three phases: phase 1, phase 2, and phase 3.

- In phase 1 clinical trials, researchers test a new drug or treatment in a small group of people for the first time to evaluate its safety, determine a safe dosage range, and identify side effects.
- In phase 2 clinical trials, the study drug or treatment is given to a larger group of people to see if it is effective and to further evaluate its safety.
- In phase 3 studies, the study drug or treatment is given to large groups of people to further determine its effectiveness, monitor side effects, compare it to commonly used treatments, and collect information that will allow the drug or treatment to be used safely.

Compared with many other disease areas, prognosis for cancer patients tends to be poorer and they generally have fewer treatment options. Therefore, clinical development of a cancer treatment is often more condensed than the typical phase 1/2/3 drug development model. In oncology, an investigational agent is usually evaluated in one or more earlier-stage trials (phases 1 and 2, involving about 20–80 patients) to determine dosing and evaluate for safety and preliminary signals of efficacy, followed by one or more late-stage trials (phases 2 and 3, involving about 40–>200 patients). The late-stage trials are randomized, meaning that the experimental agent is being compared with a "control" treatment (usually the current standard of care), and patients are randomly assigned to receive one treatment or the other. In this way, the effect of the investigational therapy can be compared with the effect of the control treatment.

To be approved for marketing, a clinical trial of an experimental treatment typically must successfully meet its primary end point(s). Depending on the type of end point used, the U.S. Food and Drug Administration (FDA) employs two approval pathways for oncology treatments: regular approval and accelerated approval. Regular approval is based on an end point that provides direct evidence of clinical benefit (e.g., OS) or on a surrogate end point (e.g., PFS) that reliably predicts clinical benefit. Accelerated approval, which is used for new treatments that provide an advantage over currently available therapy, may be based on a less established surrogate end point that is only reasonably likely to predict clinical benefit (e.g., objective response rate to treatment). Under the terms of accelerated approval, the drug manufacturer is required to conduct post-approval studies to determine if the treatment provides direct clinical benefit (e.g., improvement in OS).

In cases in which a late-stage clinical trial fails to meet its primary end point, subset analyses (either predefined or post hoc) may find evidence of benefit in a subgroup of patients. According to conventional regulatory process, a second late-stage study conducted specifically in this patient subgroup is almost always necessary to confirm the benefit observed in the first late-stage trial.

The conventional regulatory process for developing and assessing cancer treatments is largely based on evaluation of traditional chemotherapeutics. The earlier and now standard regulatory pathways have successfully introduced a formidable arsenal of treatments against both new and recurrent cancers, but have yet to license a single therapeutic cancer vaccine to date.

CHALLENGES IN CLINICAL DEVELOPMENT OF CANCER VACCINES

Longer Trials to Reach Evaluable Clinical End Points

Experimental cancer agents are often clinically evaluated in the metastatic or advanced disease setting. For many reasons, this disease setting allows for more rapid clinical development. Often this patient population has limited or no treatment options, which provides clinical, regulatory, and financial incentive for working to fill unmet medical needs. Also, patient prognosis is usually poor due to the advanced nature of disease, which allows for trials to efficiently utilize OS as an end point. The advantage of employing such an end point is twofold: Measurement is easy, accurate, and objective, and the direct clinical value of survival improvement is unquestioned. In addition, trials in the metastatic or advanced disease setting may measure effect on surrogate end points such as tumor response or time to progression, which can also be evaluated in a relatively short time frame given the high tumor burden and poor prognosis of the patient population. The long timeline required to collect data on these end points makes the newer adaptive clinical trial design, intended to accelerate clinical development by using early evaluation of incoming trial data to refine patient selection, unfeasible in these disease settings.

There are several differences between traditional cancer treatments and therapeutic cancer vaccines, which largely stem from the differences in the action of newer targeted treatments such as cancer vaccines compared with the classical, cytotoxic (cell-killing) that characterize most of the current cancer treatments. Supported by numerous animal studies, these differences are consistent with basic principles of tumor immunology, and include:

- The action of cancer vaccines is primarily cytostatic rather than cytotoxic; therefore, treatment effect typically includes slowing tumor growth instead of reducing tumor burden.
- Cancer vaccines are most effective when tumor burden is low and thus function well in the earlier-stage disease or adjuvant treatment settings.
- There appears to be a latent period before cancer vaccines exert a treatment effect. This is likely due to the time required for adequate tumor-targeting immune mechanisms to maximally expand.

Collectively, these differences translate into longer development timelines. Preclinical and clinical research strongly indicate that because of lower tumor burden, targeted treatments such as therapeutic cancer vaccines are likely to have their highest effect in earlier-stage disease or adjuvant treatment and/or in the minimal residual disease (MRD) settings. However, clinical trials involving these "better-prognosis" patients can be challenging due to the long timelines required. Because of the improved prognosis of these patient groups, collecting data on OS or recurrence-free survival—both meaningful end points in the earlier-stage or adjuvant/MRD settings—often takes many years. The lower tumor burden in these better-prognosis patients means that the "faster" end points utilized in the metastatic/advanced disease setting (e.g., tumor response, time to progression) are often not applicable. From a development standpoint, the size and duration of late-stage trials in the earlier-stage disease or adjuvant treatment setting leads to excessive expense and unusually long timelines.

Identification of Optimal Patient Population

An additional challenge in the clinical development of cancer vaccines is that— despite evidence suggesting maximum benefit in better-prognosis patients—it is impossible to precisely identify the target treatment group for any given vaccine in any given indication without conducting a large randomized trial. Because the patients' immune response is part of his own treatment and must be intact for a vaccine to work, the stage of the cancer as well as history of prior therapies are much more important considerations for therapeutic vaccines than for conventional cancer treatments. This makes the selection of a patient population especially critical. Often a vaccine's effect must be evaluated across a range of disease stages to identify exactly which stages are most responsive to the treatment. The target treatment population may vary by vaccine as well as by cancer type; therefore, a large randomized trial must be conducted for each vaccine in each indication for which it is to be developed.

According to current regulatory process, any benefit observed in a subgroup of patients—even if statistically significant in predefined or post hoc analyses—in most of the cases must be subsequently confirmed in a second randomized trial involving this subgroup. Therefore, these large, late-stage trials must be conducted sequentially, meaning that a late-stage development program could last more than 10 years, which currently represents a significant impediment to the success of the field of cancer vaccines.

Lack of Early Surrogate Markers

The lack of information with which to orient initial late-stage studies can be attributed to the absence of a reliable early marker or critical event that indicates that clinical benefit may be associated with the experimental treatment. Newer therapies such as therapeutic cancer vaccines, EGFR/HER2/neu inhibitors, and angiostatins tend to affect cancers in a different manner compared with traditional cancer treatments. They appear to slow the course of disease without causing earlier-measurable tumor shrinkage. Therefore, the effect of treatment only becomes apparent later, when the growth of the tumor lesions is retarded or absent, and the comparative time to progression is slowed. Treatment effect in the earlier-stage disease or adjuvant treatment settings can be even longer to ascertain, as the minimal tumor burden in these settings makes quicker end points such as tumor response or time to progression inapplicable. Therefore, identification of a surrogate marker or critical event indicative of clinical benefit could provide earlier feedback to help identify the group of patients most likely to benefit from treatment. This could help shorten development timelines by making the newer adaptive trial designs feasible in the earlier-disease/adjuvant treatment setting: By identifying patients that seem to be benefiting most from treatment early in patient enrollment, enrollment criteria could be tailored to focus on enrolling the optimal patient population. This could potentially eliminate the need for a second trial to confirm subset analysis findings, affording the opportunity for a single, late-stage clinical trial to establish all of the efficacy and safety information necessary to support a treatment's initial licensure.

In the metastatic disease setting, surrogate markers related to tumor response can be utilized. In the earlier-disease/adjuvant treatment setting, however, in which tumor response cannot be assessed, a reliable marker has yet to be identified. In this better-prognosis setting, there are many scientific and technological hurdles to be overcome, even ones as basic as availability of immunoassays that are amenable to routine use and can undergo adequate validation. Work continues in the development of reliable immunological biomarkers.

Following the 2006 Meeting of the Cancer Vaccine Consortium, Finke et al. identified the challenges of developing effective anticancer immunotherapies as related to the following factors: (1) underlying heterogeneity in some of the cancers and patient cohorts selected for study, (2) the longer time required to establish an effective cellular immune response versus the observation period designed into the study, and (3) diminished immunocompetence in patients with high tumor burden. Planning for phase 3 trials also encounters the difficulty that arise when using historical data to estimate the mean survival time or other end points in the control or experimental groups and aggressive projections of the ultimate benefit of active cancer immunotherapy. Finally, there is the long time and high cost of running clinical studies with cancer vaccines (31).

REGULATORY CONSIDERATIONS AND A NEW CLINICAL PARADIGM

There are a few regulatory considerations that have the opportunity to facilitate clinical development of cancer vaccines. In December 2006, the U.S. FDA issued a proposed rule to amend the regulation concerning charging patients for investigational new drugs (INDs). If the proposed role becomes effective as currently written, it will permit charging for a broader range of investigational uses than presently allowed. This allowance could provide a potential mechanism to help partially fund the necessary long and expensive late-stage trials of cancer vaccines.

A new mechanism for drug approval was recently adopted in Europe that allows for granting a conditional marketing authorization (CMA) prior to full marketing approval for a treatment that preliminarily indicates a positive risk-benefit assessment in late-stage trials. In life threatening or orphan disease settings, CMAs allow patient access to treatments that have demonstrated clinically meaningful but less statistically robust findings, which require subsequent confirmation in post-marketing trials. CMAs provide an opportunity for more comprehensive cost recovery compared with charging patients for investigational treatments.

A new development paradigm for cancer vaccines was recently proposed by the Cancer Vaccine Clinical Trial Working Group (CVCTWG), a group of more than 50 experts from academia, regulatory bodies, and the biotech/pharmaceutical industry from America and Europe (32). The authors propose a clinical development model in which therapeutic cancer vaccines are investigated in two general types of clinical studies: proof-of-principle trials and efficacy trials. Designed to account for biologic features of cancer vaccines, the proposed paradigm "supports a more flexible, expeditious, and focused clinical developmental process with early and informed decision-making through prospectively defined 'go' or 'no go' decision points, use of biologic end points, adjusted clinical end points, early use of randomized trials, and adaptive design components, where applicable." However, there remain challenges with being able to effectively apply some of these concepts in the better-prognosis patient setting. The ability to glean reliable information regarding potential efficacy at time points early in a clinical trial remains a challenge and a barrier to accelerated decision making.

Continued innovation and dialogue in the regulatory process for cancer vaccine development will be critical for the sustained investment of time, effort, and funds—without which progress in this novel and important area may never be achieved.

REFERENCES

1. Heifets L. Centennial of Metchnikoff's discovery. J Reticuloendothel Soc 1982; 31(5): 381–391.
2. Siegel JH, Janis R, Alper JC, et al. Disseminated visceral Kaposi's sarcoma. Appearance after human renal homograft operation. JAMA 1969; 207(8):1493–1496.
3. Myers BD, Kessler E, Levi J, et al. Kaposi's sarcoma in kidney transplant recipients. Arch Intern Med 1974; 133(2):307–311.
4. Penn I. Kaposi's sarcoma in organ transplant recipients: report of 20 cases. Transplantation 1979; 27(1):8–11.
5. Euvrard S, Kanitakis J, Claudy A. Skin cancers after organ transplantation. N Engl J Med 2003; 348(17):1681–1691.
6. Klein G, Sjorgen HO, Klein E, et al. Demonstration of resistance against methylcholanthrene-induced sarcomas in the primary autochthonous host. Cancer Res 1960; 20: 1561–1562.
7. Klein G. Tumor antigens. Annu Rev Microbiol 1966; 20:223–252.
8. Burnet FM. Immunological aspects of malignant disease. Lancet 1967; 1(7501): 1171–1174.
9. Burnet FM. Immunological surveillance in neoplasia. Transplant Rev 1971; 7:3–25.
10. Dunn GP, Old LJ, Schreiber RD. The immunobiology of cancer immunosurveillance and immunoediting. Immunity 2004; 21(2):137–148.
11. Stebbing J, Bower M. What can oncologists learn from HIV? Lancet Oncol 2003; 4(7): 438–445.
12. Boshoff C, Weiss R. AIDS-related malignancies. Nat Rev Cancer 2002; 2(5):373–382.
13. Portsmouth S, Stebbing J, Gill J, et al. A comparison of regimens based on nonnucleoside reverse transcriptase inhibitors or protease inhibitors in preventing Kaposi's sarcoma. AIDS 2003; 17(11):F17–F22.
14. Powles T, Thirlwell C, Nelson M, et al. Immune reconstitution inflammatory syndrome mimicking relapse of AIDS related lymphoma in patients with HIV 1 infection. Leuk Lymphoma 2003; 44(8):1417–1419.
15. Bower M, Nelson M, Young AM, et al. Immune reconstitution inflammatory syndrome associated with Kaposi's sarcoma. J Clin Oncol 2005; 23(22):5224–5228.
16. Goldman B. Cancer vaccines: finding the best way to train the immune system. J Natl Cancer Inst 2002; 94(20):1523–1526.

17. Basic concepts of immunology and neuroimmunology. Available at: http://www. medscape.com. Accessed 9/19/2007.
18. Choudhury A, Mosolits S, Kokhaei P, et al. Clinical results of vaccine therapy for cancer: learning from history for improving the future. Adv Cancer Res 2006; 95:147–202.
19. Uyl-de Groot CA, Vermorken JB, Hanna MG Jr., et al. Immunotherapy with autologous tumor cell-BCG vaccine in patients with colon cancer: a prospective study of medical and economic benefits. Vaccine 2005; 23(17–18):2379–2387.
20. AUA 2007, Poster presentation # 94680: A multicenter, randomized, Phase 3 trial of a novel autologous therapeutic vaccine (vitespen) vs. observation as adjuvant therapy in patients at high risk of recurrence after nephrectomy for renal cell carcinoma.
21. Jocham D, Richter A, Hoffmann L, et al. Adjuvant autologous renal tumour cell vaccine and risk of tumour progression in patients with renal-cell carcinoma after radical nephrectomy: phase III, randomised controlled trial. Lancet 2004; 363(9409):594–599.
22. Doehn C., Richter A., Theodor R, et al. Deutscher Krebskongress. Berlin, 22.-26.03.2006. Düsseldorf, Köln: German Medical Science; 2006. Doc OP285: Prolongation of progression-free and overall survival following an adjuvant vaccination with Reniale® in patients with non-metastatic renal cell carcinoma: Secondary analysis of a multicenter phase-III.
23. Small EJ, Schellhammer PF, Higano CS, et al. Placebo-controlled phase III trial of immunologic therapy with sipuleucel-T (APC8015) in patients with metastatic, asymptomatic hormone refractory prostate cancer. J Clin Oncol 2006; 24(19):3089–3094.
24. Dendreon. Dendreon's Second Randomized Phase 3 D9902A Trial of Provenge Extends Survival in Patients with Advanced Prostate Cancer. *Press Release, Oct. 31, 2005.* Available at: http://investor.dendreon.com/ReleaseDetail.cfm? ReleaseID=178106&Header=News. Accessed 1/15/2007.
25. Favrille announces interim analysis of secondary endpoint from pivotal phase III clinical trial of Favld following Rituxan. Favrille Press Release dated November 14, 2006 [cited 20 Apr 2007]. Available at: http://www.favrille.com. Accessed 5/31/2007.
26. Hurvitz S, Timmerman J. Recombinant, tumour-derived idiotype vaccination for indolent B cell non-Hodgkin's lymphomas: a focus on Favld. Expert Opin Biol Ther 2005; 5(6):841–852. Accessed 5/31/2007.
27. Data Safety Monitoring Board recommends continuation of MyVax® personalized immunotherapy phase III trial after second interim analysis. Press release dated July 27, 2006 [cited 10 April 2007]. Available at: www.genitope.com. Accessed 5/31/2007.
28. Biomira. Biomira announces final Phase 2b survival results of Stimuvax(R) (formerly known as BLP25 Liposome Vaccine) trial in patients with non-small cell lung cancer. Press Release, April 28, 2006. Available at: http://www.biomira.com/news/availableYears/?id=849188.
29. Butts C, Murray N, Maksymiuk A, et al. Randomized phase IIB trial of BLP25 liposome vaccine in stage IIIB and IV non-small-cell lung cancer. J Clin Oncol 2005; 23(27):6674–6681.
30. R&D Insight, Wolters Kluwer Health. Available at: http://bi.adisinsight.com. Accessed 9/19/2007.
31. Finke L, Wentworth K, Blumenstein B, et al. Lessons from Randomized Phase III Studies with Active Cancer Immunotherapies: outcomes from the 2006 Meeting of the Cancer Vaccine Consortium (CVC) 9–11 Nov, 2006, Washington, DC.
32. Hoos A, Parmiani G, Hege K, et al. A clinical development paradigm for cancer vaccines and related biologics. J Immunother 2007; 30(1):1–15.

5

Dendritic Cell Vaccines for Gliomas

Anne Luptrawan

Department of Neurosurgery, Maxine Dunitz Neurosurgical Institute, Cedars Sinai Medical Center, Los Angeles, California, U.S.A.

Gentao Liu

Division of Hematology/Oncology, Cedars Sinai Medical Center, David Geffen School of Medicine at UCLA, Los Angeles, California, U.S.A.

John S. Yu and Suzane Brian

Department of Neurosurgery, Maxine Dunitz Neurosurgical Institute, Cedars Sinai Medical Center, Los Angeles, California, U.S.A.

INTRODUCTION

The total number of new cases of primary malignant brain tumors in the United States in 2005 was 21,690 as estimated by the Central Brain Tumor Registry of the United States (CBRTUS). Astrocytomas are the most common primary brain tumor. Glioblastoma multiforme (GBM) is the most aggressive and malignant form with a median survival of only 15 months despite best possible treatment—surgical resection followed by radiation and chemotherapy. GBM can transition from a lower grade glioma (secondary GBM) or can develop de novo (primary GBM).

Despite advances in surgical technique, chemotherapy, and radiation therapy, the prognosis for patients with malignant glioma remains poor. Even after optimal treatment with surgical resection followed by chemoradiation therapy, the median survival of GBM is 15 months. The infiltrative nature of the disease, a central nervous system (CNS) microenvironment that can escape immune surveillance, and resistance of tumor to chemotherapy contribute to a grim prognosis.

Dendritic cells (DCs) have an ability to promote an effective antitumor immune response and sensitize glioma cells to chemotherapy as demonstrated in recent trials. This chapter will discuss results of recent DC-vaccine clinical trials and explore future strategies of DC vaccines for malignant gliomas.

The inherent vulnerability of the brain parenchyma and complex character of the tumor itself can explain the poor response of malignant brain tumors to current therapies (1,2). As the name implies, glioblastoma is multiform, both grossly and genetically. GBM has various deletions and amplifications, and point mutations leading to activation of signal transduction pathways downstream of tyrosine kinase receptors such as epidermal growth factor receptor (EGFR) and platelet-derived growth factor receptor (PDGFR), as well as to disruption of cell cycle–arrest pathways by *INK4a-ARF* loss or by *p53* mutations associated with CDK4 amplification or RB loss (3).

The brain's physical isolation from the systemic circulation by the blood-brain barrier (BBB), absence of lymphatic vessels, lack of resident DCs and human leukocyte antigens (HLA) on brain cells makes it an immunologically privileged organ. The neuronal environment is protected from surveillance by immune cells in part by the BBB which functions to regulate passage of macromolecules and intravascular immune cells from the lumen of vessels in the neural parenchyma into the extravascular compartment.

The location of cells within the brain is variable, making complete resection of malignant gliomas difficult (2). Tumor cells can be found centimeters away from the primary tumor site. Invasion of glioma cells into surrounding normal brain parenchyma is accomplished via white matter tracts, perivascular and periventricular spaces. In gliomatosis cerebri, cells spread diffusely and in severe cases, can involve the entire brain. Tumor cells invade critical structures creating mass effect and causing irreversible damage to areas needed for patient survival. The genetic instability, cellular heterogeneity, and disseminated nature of malignant gliomas make current treatment strategies to eliminate all residual intracranial tumor reservoirs unsuccessful (4,5a). Therefore, recurrence of tumor is inevitable and contributes to the lethality of this disease.

CELLULAR IMMUNITY

Cell-mediated immunity requires T cells to be in direct contact with their targets in order to cause injury to tumor cells. A cellular immune response is dependent on T-cell receptors' specific recognition of cell-surface antigens and its ability to recognize and destroy foreign cells, including host cells bearing intracellular pathogens. The presence of both foreign antigens and self-antigens on a cell's surface is needed to activate T cells in response to a foreign antigen. Activation of the cell-mediated immune attack triggers complementary T-cell clone proliferation and differentiation, which yields a large number of activated T cells to carry out various cell-mediated responses. Direct killing of host cells harboring mutated proteins from malignant transformations in cancer cells is done by cytotoxic T cells (killer T cells or $CD8^+$ cells) (5b).

The mechanisms designed to prevent autoimmunity protect tumors from their rejection (5b). One mechanism involved with tolerance is central tolerance. Immature T cells that would react to the body's own proteins are triggered by the thymus to undergo apoptosis (5a). Thus, the population of autoreactive T cells that survived negative selection has only low to intermediate activity to self-tumor antigens and is incapable of responding to tumor antigens with high avidity (5a). Another mechanism of tolerance is T-cell anergy or peripheral tolerance. The presence of two specific simultaneous signals, costimulatory signals from its compatible antigen and stimulatory cosignal molecule, B7, which is found only on the surface of an antigen-presenting cell (APC), is required for T-cell activation. In the absence of costimulatory molecules, T cells become anergic or inactivated if they bind to MHC: self-antigen ligands. Glioma cells express MHC: self-peptide ligands but do not express costimulatory molecules (6). Antigen plus cosignal are never present for self-antigens because these antigens are not handled by cosignal-bearing APCs. Anergic T cells do not proliferate or differentiate into armed effector cells upon recounter of self-antigen even if they receive costimulatory signals leading to tumor-specific T-cell ignorance (5a). Inhibition by Treg cells (CD4$^+$/CD25$^+$) is another mechanism by which autoreactive lymphocyte clones are inhibited. They can inhibit DC maturation and their antigen-presenting function (7) as well as T cell activation and proliferation. The mechanism of suppression by T cells is contact dependent and is often mediated by interleukin (IL)-10 and transforming growth factor-β (TGF-β) (8). Gomez and Kruse report that recently identified human CD8$^+$CD25$^+$ lymphocytes were capable of suppressing allogeneic and autologous T-cell proliferation in a cell contact–dependent manner (5a). Treg cells are elevated in the peripheral blood and tumor microenvironment in cancer patients, suggesting Treg cells may prevent the initiation of antitumor responses directed toward shared self-antigens (9).

The major histocompatibility complex (MHC) is the code for surface membrane–enclosed self-antigens (5b). MHC is a group of genes that directs the synthesis of MHC molecules, or self-antigens, which are plasma membrane–bound glycoproteins. Engulfed foreign antigens are escorted to the cell surface by MHC comolecules for presentation by APCs. T cells typically only bind with MHC self-antigens only in association with a foreign antigen such as a mutated cellular protein of a cancerous body cell. The immune system is alerted of the presence of an undesirable agent within the cell upon the combined presence of the self- and non-self-antigens displayed at the cell surface. Specific T-cell receptors fit a particular MHC–foreign antigen complex in complementary fashion. The T-cell receptor must also match the appropriate MHC protein. Cytotoxic T cells respond to foreign antigen only in association with MHC class I glycoproteins, which are found on the surface of virtually all nucleated body cells. Helper T cells respond to MHC class II glycoproteins which are found on the surface of B cells, cytotoxic T cells, and macrophages.

Immune surveillance is a process by which the T-cell system recognizes and destroys newly arisen, potentially cancerous tumor cells before they have a chance to multiply and spread. Immune surveillance against cancer depends on interplay among cytotoxic T cells, natural killer (NK) cells, macrophages, and interferon. These cells secrete interferon which functions to inhibit the division of cancer cells and amplify the immune cells' killing ability. Cancer cells have the ability to escape detection by immune mechanisms. It is believed that cancer cells fail to display identifying antigens on their surface or be surrounded by counterproductive blocking antibodies that interfere with T-cell function (5b). The coating of the tumor cells by these blocking antibodies can protect the tumor cell from attack by cytotoxic T cells. As the tumor proliferates, the tumor cells may accumulate additional mutations which may confer additional immunoevasive survival advantages on the growing neoplasm, and by the time the cancer is clinically detectable, it has developed potent immunosuppressive qualities that enable it to depress host antitumor immunity (4).

DENDRITIC CELLS

The most potent APCs are DCs. DCs have an important role in immune surveillance, antigen capture, and antigen presentation (5b). Tumor cells are known to be poor APCs. Cytotoxic T cells, as established by a strong body of evidence, play a vital role in mounting an effective antitumor immune response (10–12). The presence of a tumor antigen is necessary to generate effective tumoricidal T-cell immunity. The introduction of a naive T cell to a tumor antigen results in T-cell activation, clonal expansion, and exertion of cytolytic effector function. Patients with malignant gliomas have shown a defective antitumor immune response. Tumor cells release amplified immunosuppressive chemokines that depresses the ability of native APCs to recognize, ingest, and process tumor-derived antigens (12–14). Effective cytotoxic T-cell effector function is dependent on effective antigen presentation. Thus, the establishment of a viable immunotherapeutic approach to the treatment of malignant gliomas requires a strategy that successfully introduces tumor antigens to T cells in vivo.

A promising treatment strategy is DC-based vaccines that elicit tumor-specific antigen presentation to the immune system. Many costimulatory molecules are abundantly expressed on DCs. Effective activation of naive T cells is dependent on these costimulatory molecules that have the capacity to efficiently process and present antigenic peptides in combination with cell-surface MHC. DCs are the most potent of the APCs and are capable of initiating cytolytic T-cell function in vitro and in vivo (15). Recent advances in DC biology have allowed us to generate large number of DCs in vitro where normally, in circulation, DCs are present in very small numbers (16). Neoplastic tumors such as lymphoma, melanoma, prostate carcinoma, and renal cell carcinoma have demonstrated the ability to elicit antitumor immunity after vaccination in tumor-bearing hosts with DCs derived in vitro primed against tumor-specific antigens in culture (17–20). Siesjo was the first to demonstrate the efficacy of a peripherally administered tumor-derived peptide-pulsed DC vaccine in generating antitumor cytotoxic immunity in a rodent glioma model (21). A DC-vaccine study in melanoma demonstrated a correlation between the development of antigen-specific T-cell responses and a favorable clinical outcome (22).

IMPAIRED IMMUNE FUNCTION ASSOCIATED WITH MALIGNANT GLIOMAS

It has been demonstrated that patients diagnosed with GBM present with significant impaired immune function (23,24). The induction of potent and sustained antitumor immune responses in the immunocompetent host is extremely challenging due to intrinsic tumor tolerance mechanisms (5a). Studies have described tumor cells' ability to evade immune attack by using various strategies. Gomez and Kruse describe the various mechanisms of malignant glioma immune resistance and sources of immunosuppression (5a). We discuss their findings below.

Tumor cells produce immunosuppressive factors such as PGE2, TGF-β, and IL-10. PGE2 is a COX-2-derived prostaglandin E2 which promotes tumor cell invasion, motility, and angiogenesis upon binding to its receptor EPI-4 (5a). PGE2 also induces immunosuppression by downregulating production of T helper T_H1 cytokines (IL-2, IFN-γ, and TNF-α) and upregulating T_H2 cytokines (IL-4, IL-10, and IL-6) (25). PGE2 also inhibits T-cell activation and suppresses the antitumor activity of NK cells (26,27), and can enhance suppressive activity of Treg cells.

TGF-β is involved with regulating inflammation, angiogenesis, and proliferation (28), and is expressed by a variety of cancers including astrocytomas and appears to be the major isoform expressed by glioblastomas. TGF-β inhibits T-cell activation and proliferation (29,30), and maturation and function of professional APCs (31–33). TGF-β also inhibits synthesis of cytotoxic molecules including perforin, granzymes A and B, IFN-γ, and FasL in activated cytotoxic T-lymphocyte (CTL) (32,33). TGF-β can facilitate conversion of naive T cells to a Treg phenotype, thereby playing a role in tumor tolerance and may recruit Tregs toward the primary tumor site as a means of immune evasion (5a). IL-10 inhibits IL-2-induced T-cell proliferation (34), DC, and macrophage activation of T cells (35), and downmodulates class II MHC on APCs and is expressed by Treg cells (8) and human gliomas (35).

In order to evade immune attack, tumor cells impair the adhesive effector between tumor cell interactions and protective tumor cloaks (5a). Tumor cells develop strategies to prevent their adhesion by immune effector cells. A mechanism of evasion from tumor-specific T and NK cell lysis is disruption of leukocyte function antigen-1 (LFA-1) and intercellular adhesion molecule-1 (ICAM-1) interactions which inhibit target cell lysis (36,37).

MHC class I molecules, or HLA, are required for presentation of foreign antigen peptides to cytotoxic T cells and for the engagement of receptors that regulate NK-cell activity (38). The brain displays low or absent levels of MHC class I. Tumor cells can evade T-cell detection and subsequent induced cytotoxicity if they display aberrant HLA class I expression (5a). Complete HLA class I loss may be caused by mutations of both β_2-m alleles with the absence of β_2-m expression; HLA class I heavy chain/β_2-m/peptide complexes will not form nor be transported to the cell surface (5a).

NK cells can kill cancer cells without prior sensitization. They are responsible for killing HLA class I–deficient tumor cells (38). In neoplastic conditions, HLA class I expression is often altered, breaking NK cell tolerance (5a). Ectopic HLA-G expression is a mechanism of tumor evasion of T and NK cell lysis (39) and is believed to protect the fetus from allorejection by maternal NK and T cells (5a). HLA-G is expressed on primary GBM and by established glioma cell lines (39). HLA-G expression causes glioma cells to be resistant to alloreactive CTL lysis and its inhibitory signals are strong enough to counteract NK-activating signals.

NK and activated T cells regulate tumor growth via the Fas apoptosis pathway; however, tumor cells may disrupt this pathway at many levels within the signaling cascade (5a). Disruption of Fas-induced apoptosis or upregulation of FasL may provide tumor-cell protection to T lymphocyte–induced cell injury (5a). Decoy receptor 3 (DcR3) is expressed by brain tumors and inhibits Fas-induced apoptosis (40,41). Decreased expression of Fas or secretion of FasL decoy receptor, DcR3, by glioma cells inhibits death receptor–induced apoptosis. Tumor cells can cause T-cell apoptosis when they counterattack T cells by expressing FasL which engages Fas on the T-cell plasma membrane (5a).

DC–BASED IMMUNOTHERAPY: RESULTS OF PHASE I AND II CLINICAL TRIALS

It is very difficult to therapeutically target every remaining individual tumor cell due to the disseminated nature of GBM. It is extremely important to eliminate all intracranial neoplastic foci left behind after surgical resection of the primary tumor (4). The use of the immune system to target residual tumor cells is one such strategy to enhance visibility of tumor cells to the immune system.

In a phase I study, Yu and colleagues describe the use of a DC vaccine in patients with newly diagnosed high-grade glioma (42). After surgical resection and external-beam radiotherapy, nine patients were given a series of three DC vaccinations using DCs cultured from patients' peripheral blood mononuclear cells (PBMC) pulsed ex vivo with autologous tumor cell-surface peptide isolated by means of acid elution. Each DC vaccination was given intradermally every other week over a six-week period. Four of the nine patients who had radiological evidence of disease progression underwent repeat surgery after receiving the third vaccination. Two of the four patients who underwent re-resection had robust infiltration of CD8$^+$ and CD45RO$^+$ T cells which was not apparent in the tumor specimen resected prior to DC trial entry (Fig. 1). Comparison of long-term survival data between the study group and matched controls demonstrated an increase in median survival of 455 days versus 257 days for the control group, conferring some survival benefit after DC vaccination.

Given the promising results and absence of observed autoimmune toxicity in the phase I study, Yu and colleagues expanded the study into a phase II trial (43). Fourteen patients with recurrent (12 patients) and newly diagnosed

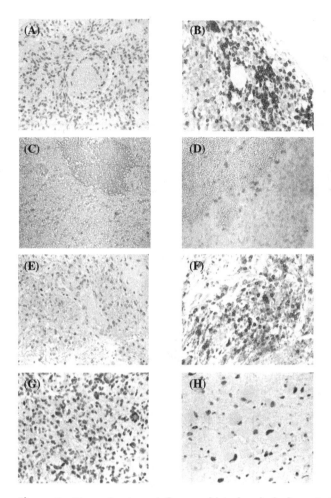

Figure 1 (*See color insert.*) **Immunohistochemical characterization of infiltrating cells in intracranial tumor before and after DC vaccination:** Intratumoral CD8+ cells, pre- (**A**), and post-vaccination (**B**). Intratumoral CD4+ cells, pre- (**C**), and post-vaccination (**D**). Intratumoral CD45RO+ cells, pre- (**E**), and post-vaccination (**F**). Intratumoral CD8+ cells pre- (**G**) and post-recurrence (**H**) in a non-vaccinated patient.

(2 patients) malignant glioma, including anaplastic astrocytoma and GBM, were given three vaccinations with autologous DC pulsed with autologous tumor lysate every other week over a six-week period. In four out of nine patients, as part of an HLA-restricted tetramer staining assay, it was found that there were one or more tumor-associated antigen (TAA)-specific CTL clones against melanoma antigen-encoding gene-1, gp100, and human epidermal growth factor receptor (HER)-2 (Fig. 2). DC vaccination offered a significant survival benefit

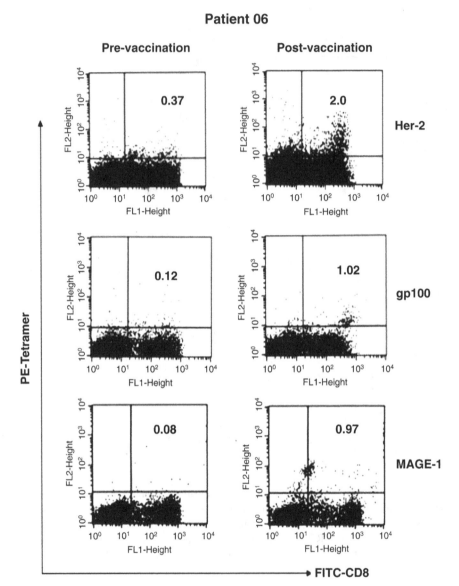

Figure 2 **Representative flow cytometry plots from a single glioma patient vaccinated with autologous tumor lysate pulsed DCs.** PBMC isolated pre- (left column) and post-vaccination (right column) were stained with HLA restricted tetramers for HER-2, gp100, and MAGE-1 (*y*-axis). Additionally, cells were stained for the CD8 antigen (*x*-axis). Plots indicate a significant increase in the number of cells that registered as double positive (i.e. bound to antigen specific tetramers and positive for CD8). This demonstrates an expansion in the populations of CTL specific for these TAAs in this patient following DC vaccination.

as evidenced by an increase in median survival of 133 weeks for the study group versus 30 weeks for the control group.

In a phase I study by Kikuchi and colleagues (44), eight patients were treated with a series of three to seven intradermal vaccinations with DC-autologous glioma fusion cells. Glioma fusion cells were used as a strategy to improve DC-mediated TAA presentation by enhancing tumor cell–DC interaction. Although the ability to induce a tumor-specific immune response was demonstrated, only slight temporary responses to therapy were detected in two patients who had tumor progression on follow-up neuroimaging studies.

Kikuchi and colleagues reported a clinical trial using DC-glioma fusion cells and recombinant human IL-12 (45) after a mouse brain tumor model demonstrated systemic administration of recombinant IL-12 enhanced antitumor effect of this vaccine (46). The trial involved 15 patients who received vaccine therapy after progression of disease despite standard chemotherapy and/or radiation therapy. The vaccine of DC-autologous glioma fusion cells was given intradermally close to a cervical lymph node followed by recombinant IL-12 (30 ng/kg) injected subcutaneously at the same site on days 3 and 7. Two six-week courses of this regimen were completed with the second course starting two to five weeks after the last dose of IL-12.

However, results of this trial demonstrated limited success of the DC-glioma fusion cell vaccine. Only two patients demonstrated significant increase in cytolytic activity after vaccination, as shown in a Cr-releasing cytolytic assay (13) using peripheral blood lymphocytes and autologous glioma cells. Cytolytic activity was almost nonexistent in the remainder of patients in the study group. CD4$^+$ T-cell subsets were not observed, although CD8$^+$ T-cell infiltration was more robust in recurrent tumor specimens, with pathologic findings of larger tumor cells containing multiple nuclei and wide cytoplasm, when compared to primary tumors. Failure of tumor-specific T-helper 1 induction and/or the existence of tolerogenic CD4$^+$ T-cell subsets may be a reason for the limited success of the DC-glioma fusion cell vaccine. The potential for T-helper 1 and resident APCs to stimulate each other lends to support TAA-specific CTL responses. The development of a successful antiglioma vaccine may depend on the helper activity of the antigen-specific T-helper subset which can interact with APCs to activate them in the tumor microenvironment (47).

A direct injection of DCs into tumor is a novel immunotherapeutic approach. DCs acquire and process tumor antigens in situ allowing migration to regional lymphoid organs via lymphoid vessels thereby initiating significant tumor-specific immune responses in the CNS (12,48). Yamanaka and colleagues described results of a phase I/II clinical trial in which five glioma patients received intradermal vaccination of autologous tumor lysate–pulsed DC vaccination, whereas another five patients underwent intratumoral injection of autologous immature DCs in addition to intradermal vaccination of tumor lysate–pulsed DCs (49). This study used immature DCs since the ability to capture, process, and traffic antigens have been demonstrated by DCs only in their immature state (50). Patients who received both the intratumoral and the intradermal vaccines demonstrated reduction in the size of contrast-enhancing tumor on neuroimaging. This indicates that immature DCs injected intratumorally can potentially induce an antitumor immune response by their ability to capture and process TAAs in situ. For patients with surgically unresectable tumors not allowing for sufficient tumor specimen and/or recurrent gliomas, this may be a novel strategy.

In a subsequent phase I/II clinical study, Yamanaka and colleagues, describe the clinical evaluation of malignant glioma patients vaccinated with DCs pulsed by an autologous tumor lysate (51). Twenty-four patients with malignant glioma (6 grade III malignant gliomas and 18 grade IV GBM) status postsurgical resection of tumor, external beam radiation therapy, and nitrosourea-based chemotherapy were enrolled in this study. These patients were monitored for recurrence via brain imaging (MRI or CT), and upon evidence of tumor recurrence, DC immunotherapy was initiated. Twelve patients received maintenance glucocorticoid therapy with prednisone 30 mg/day during DC therapy.

DCs were injected intradermally close to a cervical lymph node, or intradermally and intratumorally via an Ommaya reservoir. Patients received DC pulsed with autologous tumor lysate every 3 weeks and continued with up to 10 vaccinations depending on the clinical response. The mean number of administrations was 7.4 times intradermally and 4.6 times intratumorally. In the phase I section of the protocol, 17 patients received administration of immatured DCs pulsed by tumor lysate intradermally or both intradermally and intratumorally. Of the 17 patients, 2 had minor response, 6 had no change, and 9 had progressive disease. In the phase II section of the protocol, seven patients received administration of DCs matured with OK-432 pulsed by tumor lysate given intradermally and immatured DCs given intratumorally via an Ommaya reservoir. One out of the seven patients had partial response, one had minor response, four had no change, and one had progressive disease on MRI. Yamanaka and colleagues found that those 7 patients with GBM who received DCs matured with OK-432 had a significantly increased overall survival compared to the 11 patients who received DCs without OK-432 maturation. They also found that the GBM patients that received both intratumoral and intradermal DC vaccinations had a longer overall survival time than the patients who received intradermal administration alone. Survival of 18 DC-vaccinated patients was compared to 27 nonselected age-, gender-, and disease-matched controls that similarly underwent surgical resection, radiation, and nitrosourea-based chemotherapy. In the DC vaccinated group, results demonstrated a median overall survival time of 480 days with a percentage of overall survival 23.5% at 2 years versus 400 days in the control group with a percentage of overall survival 3.7% at 2 years, conferring DC vaccination is associated with prolonged survival.

In a phase I, dose-escalation study, Liau and colleagues enrolled 12 patients with GBM (7 newly diagnosed, 5 recurrent) and treated them with 1, 5, or 10 million autologous DCs pulsed with acid-eluted autologous tumor peptides (52). The newly diagnosed patients underwent surgical resection followed by standard external beam radiation therapy and then administration of DC vaccinations. The recurrent patients had undergone radiation therapy and/or chemotherapy previously before presenting with recurrent tumor and then underwent surgical resection before administration of DC vaccines. After DC vaccination for all 12 GBM patients, overall survival was 100% at six months, 75% at one year, and 50% at 2 years with two long-term survivors ($\geq$4 years). Median time to progression was 15.5 months and median overall survival was 23.4 months. For those five patients with ongoing progressive disease and bulky tumor, median overall survival was 11.7 months. For the seven patients with either gross stable disease or no measurable residual disease at baseline, overall survival was 18 to over 58 months. This resulted in an overall median survival benefit of 35.8 months after DC vaccination when compared to control population who had a median overall survival of 18.3 months.

Postvaccination using conventional CTL assays, six patients were found to have peripheral tumor-specific CTL activity. These patients did not have peripheral CTL activity prior to vaccination. Those who developed systemic antitumor cytotoxicity had longer survival time compared to those patients who did not. All of the patients who had stable/minimal residual disease at baseline generated a positive CTL response (100%), whereas those with active progressive disease at baseline did not produce statistically significant cell-mediated CTL responses (0%), suggesting that those with active tumor progression/recurrence may have an impaired ability to mount an effective cellular antitumor immune response. Eight patients who developed tumor progression on follow-up MRI postvaccine therapy underwent repeat surgical resection or biopsy. A robust infiltration of CD3$^+$ tumor-infiltrating lymphocytes (TIL), not present in tissue samples taken prior to DC vaccination, was found in four of the eight patients who survived >30 months. However, those patients who died within one year (3 patients) demonstrated no significant infiltration, demonstrating that accumulation of tumor-specific T cells locally within tumors is associated with positive clinical responses. CD8$^+$/CD45RO$^+$ memory T cells with lesser number of CD4$^+$ helper T cells were the majority of TILs identified.

Liau and colleagues also found that patients who had minimal tumor burden prevaccination (4 of 4) demonstrated evidence of increased TIL, whereas those with progressive disease prevaccination (3 of 3) showed no detectable increase in TIL. The authors suggest that clinical benefit from DC vaccination may be limited by active tumor recurrence and/or bulky residual tumor, which can negatively influence T lymphocytes' ability to accumulate within the local tumor microenvironment. This study also looked at expression of TGF-β_2 and IL-10 using reverse transcription-PCR and immunohistochemistry in the tumor tissue to demonstrate whether secretion of immunosuppressive cytokines by the tumors affected local accumulation of T cells. They found that those patients with detectable TIL had lower quantitative expression of TGF-β_2 and had a longer survival (>30 months) than those with higher quantitative expression of TGF-β_2. The authors suggest that a high expression of TGF-β_2 may decrease the ability of TIL to accumulate within CNS gliomas to mount a clinical relevant local antitumor immune response in brain cancer patients.

MALIGNANT GLIOMAS AND CHEMORESISTANCE

Despite recent advances in surgery, chemotherapy, and radiation therapy, the increases in median survival in patients with GBM remain modest. With best-known treatment, the median survival for GBM is currently increased to just two to three months. A major reason for this modest response to therapy is chemotherapy resistance by malignant tumor cells. Resistance to chemotherapy can be due to either an innate property of malignant tumor cells or their ability to acquire resistance during drug treatment. Over the past decade, researchers have begun to pave the road to understanding the molecular mechanisms by which brain tumor cells develop a drug-resistant phenotype with much success (53). Fas antigen (FasA) and Fas ligand has been shown to participate in cytotoxicity mediated by T lymphocytes and NK cells. By using the combination of anti-Fas Ab and various drugs, Wakahara and his colleagues in 1997 demonstrated the ability to overcome drug resistance in ovarian cancer (54). In animal models, efficient elimination of both intrinsically resistant myeloma cells and acquired multiple drug-resistant (MDR) tumor cells was shown with granulocyte-macrophage colony-stimulating factor (GM-CSF)- and IL-12-expressing tumor cell vaccines (55). Drug-resistant tumors are probably more readily lysed by MHC-restricted, tumor-associated CTLs as some drug-resistant tumor cells expressed significant higher HLA class I–surface antigens and TAP mRNA than drug-sensitive cells (56,57). Extensive investigations of intracellular vaccinations targeting molecules related to drug resistance have been performed (58). Through collective evidence, immunotherapy is demonstrating to be an effective approach in overcoming a major treatment barrier in cancer treatment—drug resistance with chemotherapy. Many cancer immunotherapy trials are limited in demonstrating an effective antitumor immune response. However, newer DC-based therapy approaches have demonstrated some success. Liu and his colleagues demonstrated for the first time that targeting of tumor-associated antigen TRP-2 by DC vaccination significantly increased chemotherapeutic sensitivity. Immunotherapy not only induces T-cell cytotoxicity as is well established, but can also make tumors more sensitive to drug therapy (59).

SENSITIZATION TO CHEMOTHERAPY OF GLIOMA CELLS AFTER DC THERAPY

It was demonstrated by Fisk in 1998 that by eliminating tumor cells expressing higher levels of MHC class I and relevant tumor antigens by co-culturing tumor cells with CTLs, CTL-resistant tumor cells exhibited increased drug sensitivity (57). Liu and colleagues recently found that significant drug resistance to carboplatin and temozolomide compared to wild-type U-373 (W-U373) resulted

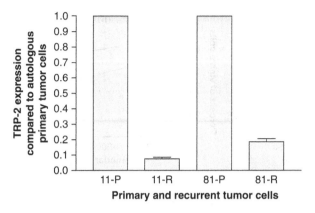

Figure 3 TRP-2 expression in primary (P) and recurrent (R) tumor cells. Total RNA was extracted from tumor cells derived from patient No. 81 and patient No. 11. TRP-2 mRNA expression was measured by real-time qPCR. The expression was firstly normalized by internal control B-actin. The relative TRP-2 mRNA level of recurrent tumor was presented as the fold decrease compared to autologous primary tumor cells. (Reproduced from Liu G. *et al.* Oncogene, 2005, 24: 5226–5234)

from the TRP-2 transfected cell line (TRP-2-U373). After immunoselection by TRP-2-specific CTL clone, CTL-resistant tumor cells (IS-TRP-2-373) developed significant increased sensitivity to carboplatin and temozolomide compared to W-U373 (59). In a phase I DC vaccination clinical trial by Liu and colleagues, TRP-2-specific cytotoxic T-cell activity was detected in patients' PBMC after active immunotherapy against unselected glioma antigens using tumor lysate–loaded DCs (60). Tumor-cell specimens were taken from postvaccination resections from two patients who developed CTL to TRP-2. Compared to autologous cell lines derived from prevaccination resections in two patients who demonstrated CTL response to TRP-2, these specimens demonstrated significantly lower TRP-2 expression (Fig. 3) and higher drug sensitivity to carboplatin and temozolomide (Fig. 4). Thus, targeting TRP-2 may provide a new strategy in improving chemotherapy sensitivity. However, not all forms of drug resistance in tumor cells develop with TRP-2. Other drug resistance–related proteins, such as EGFR, MDR-1, MRPs, HER-2, and survivin, etc., may also decrease after DC vaccination.

Another mechanism that may contribute to the sensitization of tumor cells to chemotherapy after vaccination is loss of chromosomal arms 1p and 19q. A unique constellation of molecular changes have been identified in prior studies including allelic loss of chromosome 1p and coincidental loss of chromosomal arms 1p and 19q (frequency: 50–70%), which in some gliomas, particularly in anaplastic and nonanaplastic oligodendroglioma, strongly predicts a far greater likelihood of chemotherapeutic response (61–63). For example, in a series of 55 grade II and III oligodendrogliomas, the principal independent predictor of

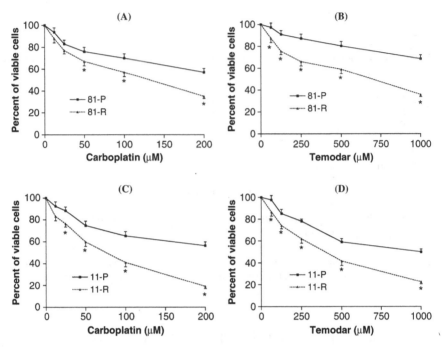

Figure 4 Drug sensitivity of in primary (P) and recurrent (R) tumor cells. Tumor cells derived from patient No. 81 and patient No. 11 were treated with various concentrations of (**A and B**) carboplatin; (**C and D**) temozolomide for 48 hours. * in the figure indicates $p < 0.05$ compared to autologous primary tumor cells. Data are from three independent experiments. (Reproduced from Liu G. *et al.* Oncogene, 2005, 24: 5226–5234)

progression-free survival after chemotherapy with procarbazine, lomustine, and vincristine plus radiotherapy was loss of heterozygosity (LOH) of chromosome 1p: median progression-free survival for 19 patients whose tumors retained both copies of 1p was only 6 months compared to 36 patients whose tumors had lost 1p alleles was 55 months (61). In a subset of high-grade gliomas, particularly in anaplastic oligodendrogliomas, specific molecular genomic changes may prove useful as markers of relative chemosensitivity. Laser-dissected pre- and post-vaccine pathological specimens were analyzed for LOH at the chromosomal loci of tumor DNA (63). This analysis revealed that after DC vaccination of young (responsive; <55 yr) patients, a prominent change in allelic loss frequency was localized to chromosomal region 1p36: 100% of patients' tumors exhibited 1p36 LOH after vaccination, whereas only 33% of patients' tumor exhibited 1p36 LOH prior to vaccination ($n = 6$) (64). The current studies utilizing DC active immunotherapy to elicit fundamental physiological changes have demonstrated the potential of improving chemosensitivity of GBMs.

MALIGNANT GLIOMA RESPONSIVENESS TO
CHEMOTHERAPY POST-DC VACCINATION

The processes that can explain a reason why tumor recurs despite CTL induction by DC vaccination are immunoselection and immunoediting. These processes allow tumor cells to escape from CTLs by antigen loss (65,66). The potential synergies between immunotherapy and other therapies must therefore be investigated due to the clinical inconsistency of cancer vaccines and the effects of immunoselection on tumor evolution (67–69). Cedars-Sinai Medical Center (68) and Brigham and Women's Hospital have conducted clinical trials to examine the synergy of vaccines with chemotherapy treatment (70). A retrospective analysis of clinical outcomes (survival and progression times) in 25 vaccinated (13 with and 12 without subsequent chemotherapy) and 13 non-vaccinated de novo GBM patients receiving chemotherapy was performed. Patients who received post-vaccine chemotherapy demonstrated longer survival times and significantly longer times to tumor recurrence after chemotherapy relative to their own previous recurrence times, as well as to patients receiving vaccine or chemotherapy alone (Fig. 5). Two of these patients who underwent

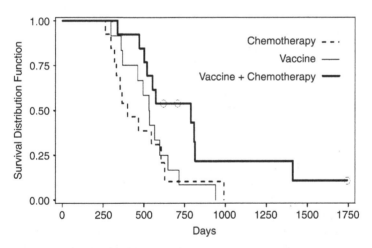

Figure 5 Overall survival in vaccine, chemotherapy, and vaccine + chemotherapy groups. Overall survival was defined as the time from first diagnosis of brain tumor (*de novo* GBM in all cases) to death due to tumor progression. Kaplan-Meier survival plots with censored values in *open circles* are shown for each group. Survival of the vaccine group was identical to that of chemotherapy group ($P = 0.7$, log-rank test). Survival of vaccine + chemotherapy group was significantly greater relative to survival in the other two groups together ($P = 0.048$, log-rank test), greater than survival in the chemotherapy group alone ($P = 0.028$, log-rank test), and greater than survival in the vaccine group alone ($P = 0.048$, log-rank test). Two of the three patients exhibiting objective tumor regression survived for >2 years (730 days) after diagnosis. (Reproduced from Wheeler CJ. *et al.* Clinical Cancer Research, 2004, 10(16): 5316–5326)

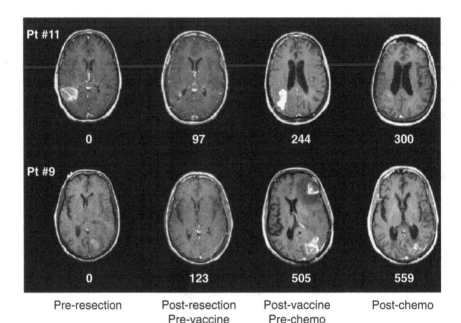

Pre-resection   Post-resection   Post-vaccine   Post-chemo
                       Pre-vaccine   Pre-chemo

Figure 6   Tumor regression following post-vaccine chemotherapy. Relative days after diagnosis are represented by the *numbers* under individual MRI scans, with individual patient scans in each row. Patient 11 recurred 82 days after vaccine initiation; patient 9 recurred 147 days after vaccine initiation, was treated surgically, and recurred 227 additional days (374 days total) after vaccine initiation. (Reproduced from Wheeler CJ. *et al.* Clinical Cancer Research, 2004, 10(16): 5316–5326)

treatment with temozolomide after recurrence demonstrated a dramatic response (Fig. 6). DC vaccination works in synergy with subsequent chemotherapy to elicit tangible clinical benefits for GBM patients. This is based on the evidence that DC vaccination induces specific CTL targeting of drug resistance–related TAAs and clinical observations. The results of these recent clinical trials strongly support the concept of utilization of DC immunotherapy to sensitize tumor cells to chemotherapy.

FUTURE STRATEGIES FOR DC VACCINES

The success of vaccines depends on the identification of appropriate tumor antigens, establishment of effective immunization strategies, and their ability to circumvent inhibitory immune mechanisms. The challenge for scientists in the future will be to further extend our fundamental knowledge of DC immunobiology, tumor immunology, and cancer biology, and to implement these findings in the rational design of DC immunotherapy for the treatment of cancer patients.

The challenge with vaccination strategies is to break tolerance so that the patient's immune system recognizes cancer cells. Several aspects involving DC vaccines need to be optimized to include the protocol of DC generation, DC subtype, dose and timing interval of vaccination, route of administration, approaches of antigen loading, and especially DC maturation (71). Recently, a group of researchers has identified a small population of cancer stem cells in adult and pediatric brain tumors (72). These cancer stem cells form neurospheres and possess the capacity for self-renewal (72). They also express genes associated with neural stem cells (NSCs) and differentiate into phenotypically diverse populations including neuronal, astrocytic, and oligodendroglial cells (73–76). Cancer stem cells are likely to share many of the properties of normal stem cells that provide for a long life span, including relative quiescence, resistance to drugs and toxins through the expression of several ABC transporters, an active DNA-repair capacity, and resistance to apoptosis. Clinically, it is observed that tumors respond to chemotherapies only to recur with renewed resilience and aggression. Although chemotherapy kills most of the cells in a tumor, cancer stem cells may be left behind which allow recurrence of tumor. Recent studies suggest that CD133$^+$ cancer stem cells are resistant to current chemotherapy (77,78) and radiation therapy (79). However, cancer stem–like cells (CSCs) could be a novel target for DC immunotherapy. More recently, Pellegatta and his colleagues have reported that that neurospheres enriched in CSCs are highly effective in eliciting a DC-mediated immune response against malignant GL261 glioma cells. These findings suggest that DC targeting of CSCs provides a higher level of protection against GL261 gliomas (80). Future vaccination therapies may be directly driven toward CSC lysates or specific tumor antigens of CSCs to improve and ameliorate the DC-vaccine efficacy (mostly evaluated as overall survival) (81).

Moreover, the effects of immunotherapy depend on the development of antigen-specific memory CD8$^+$ T cells that can express cytokines and kill antigen-bearing cells when they encounter the tumor. The induction of specific CD8$^+$-mediated antitumor immunity by DC vaccine involves the following six steps: (i) antigen threshold, (ii) antigen presentation, (iii) T-cell response, (iv) T-cell traffic, (v) target destruction, and (vi) generation of memory. Each of these steps could be significantly impacted by chemotherapy (82). Cytotoxic chemotherapy can be integrated with tumor vaccines using unique doses and schedules to break down the barriers to cancer immunotherapy, releasing the full potential of the antitumor immune response to eradicate disease. The development of new protocols by combining chemotherapy with immunotherapy to achieve therapeutic synergy will be applicable to many cancer types (83). Furthermore, synergistic effects of DC immunotherapy followed by chemotherapy have also been observed. Sensitization of malignant glioma to chemotherapy through DC vaccination provides a novel strategy to overcome the immune escape of cancer cells by immunoediting (66,71).

Finally, tumor cells can actively downregulate antitumor immunity and even create a state of immunologic unresponsiveness or self-tolerance to tumor

(*text continues on page 104*)

Table 1 Summary of results of phase I and phase II DC-based immunotherapy for malignant gliomas

Senior investigator/ reference	Trial phase	Patient population	Target disease	Vaccine	Results	Response postvaccination	Intratumoral T cells postvaccination on reoperation
Yu et al. (2001) (42)	Phase I	9 (7 GBM-N, 2 AA-N)	Newly diagnosed HGG	DC-pulsed tumor lysate, 3 biweekly vaccinations over 6-week period	Median survival of 455 days (study group) versus 257 days (control group)	4 of 7 patients elicited systemic T-cell cytotoxicity	2 of 4 patients elicited robust intratumoral cytotoxic (CD8$^+$) and memory (CD45RO$^+$) T-cell infiltration
Yu et al. (2004) (43)	Phase I	14 (3 AA, 9 GBM, 1 GBM-N, 1 AA-N)	Recurrent HGG	DC-pulsed tumor lysate, 3 biweekly vaccinations over 6-week period	Recurrent GBM ($n = 8$) 133 weeks versus 30 weeks for 26 control patients	6 of 10 patients elicited robust systemic cytotoxicity	3 of 6 patients elicited robust CD8$^+$ T-cell infiltration intratumorally
Kikuchi et al. (2001) (44)	Phase I	8 (Malignant glioma)	HGG	DC-autologous glioma fusion cells, Intradermal injections given intradermally every 3 weeks for minimum of 3 and maximum of 7 immunizations		Percentage of CD16$^+$ and CD56$^+$ cells in peripheral blood monocytes slightly increased after immunization in 4 out of 5 cases tested	
Kikuchi et al. (2004) (45)	Phase I	15 (Malignant glioma)	Recurrent HGG	DC autologous glioma fusion cells injected intradermally followed by recombinant IL-12 (30 ng/kg) for week courses	50% reduction in tumor size on magnetic resonance imaging in patients	2 of 15 patients demonstrated significant cytolytic activity	

Yamanaka et al. (2003) (49)	Phase I/II	10 (7 GBM, 3 AA)	Recurrent HGG	DC-pulsed tumor lysate every 3 weeks for a minimum of one and maximum of 10 vaccinations injected intradermally close to a cervical lymph node and/or intratumorally via an Ommaya reservoir	Increased percentage of CD56$^+$ cells in PBL after vaccination	2 patients after reoperation after vaccination demonstrated intratumoral CD4$^+$ and CD8$^+$ T-cell infiltration
					2 patients after vaccination had increase in T cells reactive against tumor lysate–pulsed DCs	
					3 patients after vaccination demonstrated only weak T-cell responses against tumor lysate–pulsed DCs	
					Those who received both intradermal and intratumoral administration ($n = 5$) demonstrated a clinical response	

(Continued)

Table 1 Summary of results of phase I and phase II DC-based immunotherapy for malignant gliomas (*Continued*)

Senior investigator/ reference	Trial phase	Patient population	Target disease	Vaccine	Results	Response postvaccination	Intratumoral T cells postvaccination on reoperation
Yamanaka et al. (2005) (51)	Phase I/II	24 (6 AA, 18 GBM) Phase I (n = 17) Phase II (n = 7)	Recurrent HGG	Upon recurrence, phase I–immatured DC-pulsed tumor lysate intradermally or both intradermally and intratumorally (via Ommaya reservoir), Phase II–matured DC (matured with OK-432)-pulsed tumor lysate intradermally administered and immature DC were intratumorally administered	GBM 480 days (study group) versus 400 days (control group) Longer survival in patients with matured DC administration Patients with both intradermal and intratumoral administration had longer survival than with intradermal alone	T cells reactive against tumor lysate–pulsed DCs increased in 7 of 24 patients after vaccination	

| Liau et al. (2005) (52). | Phase I | 12 (5 GBM, 7 GBM-N) | GBM | DC-pulsed tumor lysate, 3 biweekly intradermal vaccinations | Those who developed systemic antitumor cytotoxicity had significantly longer survival than those who did not 50% overall 2-year survival | 6 of 12 patients developed measurable systemic antitumor CTL response 1 patient had near-complete regression of residual tumor on MRI Only those with low expression of TGF-β2 and absence of bulky actively progressing tumor demonstrated intratumoral T-cell accumulation | 4 of 8 patients showed increased intratumoral infiltration by cytotoxic T cells upon reoperation after vaccination |

Abbreviations: GBM, glioblastoma multiforme; AA, anaplastic astrocytoma; RT, radiation therapy; N, newly diagnosed; EBRT, external beam radiation therapy; PBL, peripheral blood lymphocytes; MRI, magnetic resonance imaging.

antigens (84,85). Moreover, in tumor-associated lymph nodes, CD4$^+$CD25$^+$ regulatory phenotype [regulatory T cells (Tregs)] can be found which can actively suppress DC function (86). Recently, a specific subgroup of T cells (CD8$^+$ RTEs) was demonstrated to be responsive to tumor antigen and underlie age-dependent glioma clinical outcome (60). Within all GBM patients receiving post-vaccine chemotherapy, however, CD8$^+$ RTEs predicted significantly longer chemotherapeutic responses, revealing a strong link between the predominant T-cell effectors in GBM and tumor chemosensitivity. These important findings have led us to a clear future direction in the pursuit of more effective DC-vaccine glioma therapy. Any approaches including use of growth factors, hormones, adjuvants, and chemotherapeutical agents to increase newly produced CD8$^+$ RTEs and/or deplete or decrease the number of Tregs will enhance therapeutic responses and patient survival after vaccination. These concepts have undergone testing in animal models and clinical trials.

REFERENCES

1. Vescovi AL, Galli R, Reynolds BA. Brain tumour stem cells. Nat Rev Cancer 2006; 6:425–436.
2. Holland EC. Glioblastoma multiforme: the terminator. Proc Natl Acad Sci USA 2000; 97:6242–6244.
3. James CD, Olson JJ. Molecular genetics and molecular biology advances in brain tumors. Curr Opin Oncol 1996; 8:188–195.
4. Ehtesham M, Black KL, Yu JS. Recent progress in immunotherapy for malignant glioma: treatment strategies and results from clinical trials. Cancer Control 2004; 11:192–207.
5a. Gomez GG, Kruse CA. Mechanisms of malignant glioma immune resistance and sources of immunosuppression. Gene Ther Mol Biol 2006; 10:133–146.
5b. Sherwood L. The Body Defenses. In: Human physiology: from cells to systems. Fourth ed. Pacific Grove: Brooks/Cole 2001; 389–432.
6. Wintterle S, Schreiner B, Mitsdoerffer M, et al. Expression of the B7-related molecule B7-H1 by glioma cells: a potential mechanism of immune paralysis. Cancer Res 2003; 63:7462–7467.
7. Misra N, Bayry J, Lacroix-Desmazes S, et al. Cutting edge: human CD4+CD25+ T cells restrain the maturation and antigen-presenting function of dendritic cells. J Immunol 2004; 172:4676–4680.
8. Sakaguchi S. Naturally arising Foxp3-expressing CD25+CD4+ regulatory T cells in immunological tolerance to self and non-self. Nat Immunol 2005; 6:345–352.
9. Woo EY, Chu CS, Goletz TJ, et al. Regulatory CD4(+)CD25(+) T cells in tumors from patients with early-stage non-small cell lung cancer and late-stage ovarian cancer. Cancer Res 2001; 61:4766–4772.
10. Holladay FP, Lopez G, De M, et al. Generation of cytotoxic immune responses against a rat glioma by in vivo priming and secondary in vitro stimulation with tumor cells. Neurosurgery 1992; 30:499–504; discussion 504–505.
11. Dermime S, Armstrong A, Hawkins RE, et al. Cancer vaccines and immunotherapy. Br Med Bull 2002; 62:149–162.

12. Kikuchi T, Akasaki Y, Abe T, et al. Intratumoral injection of dendritic and irradiated glioma cells induces anti-tumor effects in a mouse brain tumor model. Cancer Immunol Immunother 2002; 51:424–430.

13. Zou JP, Morford LA, Chougnet C, et al. Human glioma-induced immunosuppression involves soluble factor(s) that alters monocyte cytokine profile and surface markers. J Immunol 1999; 162:4882–4892.

14. Reddy PS, Sakhuja K, Ganesh S, et al. Sustained human factor VIII expression in hemophilia A mice following systemic delivery of a gutless adenoviral vector. Mol Ther 2002; 5:63–73.

15. Banchereau J, Steinman RM. Dendritic cells and the control of immunity. Nature 1998; 392:245–252.

16. Thurner B, Roder C, Dieckmann D, et al. Generation of large numbers of fully mature and stable dendritic cells from leukapheresis products for clinical application. J Immunol Methods 1999; 223:1–15.

17. Hsu FJ, Benike C, Fagnoni F, et al. Vaccination of patients with B-cell lymphoma using autologous antigen-pulsed dendritic cells. Nat Med 1996; 2:52–58.

18. Kugler A, Stuhler G, Walden P, et al. Regression of human metastatic renal cell carcinoma after vaccination with tumor cell-dendritic cell hybrids. Nat Med 2000; 6:332–336.

19. Nestle FO, Alijagic S, Gilliet M, et al. Vaccination of melanoma patients with peptide- or tumor lysate-pulsed dendritic cells. Nat Med 1998; 4:328–332.

20. Tjoa BA, Simmons SJ, Bowes VA, et al. Evaluation of phase I/II clinical trials in prostate cancer with dendritic cells and PSMA peptides. Prostate 1998; 36:39–44.

21. Siesjo P, Visse E, Sjogren HO. Cure of established, intracerebral rat gliomas induced by therapeutic immunizations with tumor cells and purified APC or adjuvant IFN-gamma treatment. J Immunother Emphasis Tumor Immunol 1996; 19:334–345.

22. Banchereau J, Palucka AK, Dhodapkar M, et al. Immune and clinical responses in patients with metastatic melanoma to CD34(+) progenitor-derived dendritic cell vaccine. Cancer Res 2001; 61:6451–6458.

23. Brooks WH, Netsky MG, Normansell DE, et al. Depressed cell-mediated immunity in patients with primary intracranial tumors. Characterization of a humoral immunosuppressive factor. J Exp Med 1972; 136:1631–1647.

24. Young HF, Sakalas R, Kaplan AM. Inhibition of cell-mediated immunity in patients with brain tumors. Surg Neurol 1976; 5:19–23.

25. Wang D, Dubois RN. Prostaglandins and cancer. Gut 2006; 55:115–122.

26. Baxevanis CN, Reclos GJ, Gritzapis AD, et al. Elevated prostaglandin E2 production by monocytes is responsible for the depressed levels of natural killer and lymphokine-activated killer cell function in patients with breast cancer. Cancer 1993; 72:491–501.

27. Chemnitz JM, Driesen J, Classen S, et al. Prostaglandin E2 impairs CD4+ T cell activation by inhibition of lck: implications in Hodgkin's lymphoma. Cancer Res 2006; 66:1114–1122.

28. Govinden R, Bhoola KD. Genealogy, expression, and cellular function of transforming growth factor-beta. Pharmacol Ther 2003; 98:257–265.

29. Gorelik L, Flavell RA. Abrogation of TGFbeta signaling in T cells leads to spontaneous T cell differentiation and autoimmune disease. Immunity 2000; 12:171–181.

30. Ranges GE, Figari IS, Espevik T, et al. Inhibition of cytotoxic T cell development by transforming growth factor beta and reversal by recombinant tumor necrosis factor alpha. J Exp Med 1987; 166:991–998.
31. Letterio JJ, Roberts AB. Regulation of immune responses by TGF-beta. Annu Rev Immunol 1998; 16:137–161.
32. Smyth MJ, Strobl SL, Young HA, et al. Regulation of lymphokine-activated killer activity and pore-forming protein gene expression in human peripheral blood CD8+ T lymphocytes. Inhibition by transforming growth factor-beta. J Immunol 1991; 146:3289–3297.
33. Thomas DA, Massague J. TGF-beta directly targets cytotoxic T cell functions during tumor evasion of immune surveillance. Cancer Cell 2005; 8:369–380.
34. Grutz G. New insights into the molecular mechanism of interleukin-10-mediated immunosuppression. J Leukoc Biol 2005; 77:3–15.
35. Hishii M, Nitta T, Ishida H, et al. Human glioma-derived interleukin-10 inhibits antitumor immune responses in vitro. Neurosurgery 1995; 37:1160–1166; discussion 1166–1167.
36. Fiore E, Fusco C, Romero P, et al. Matrix metalloproteinase 9 (MMP-9/gelatinase B) proteolytically cleaves ICAM-1 and participates in tumor cell resistance to natural killer cell-mediated cytotoxicity. Oncogene 2002; 21:5213–5223.
37. Schiltz PM, Gomez GG, Read SB, et al. Effects of IFN-gamma and interleukin-1beta on major histocompatibility complex antigen and intercellular adhesion molecule-1 expression by 9L gliosarcoma: relevance to its cytolysis by alloreactive cytotoxic T lymphocytes. J Interferon Cytokine Res 2002; 22:1209–1216.
38. O'Connor GM, Hart OM, Gardiner CM. Putting the natural killer cell in its place. Immunology 2006; 117:1–10.
39. Wiendl H, Mitsdoerffer M, Hofmeister V, et al. A functional role of HLA-G expression in human gliomas: an alternative strategy of immune escape. J Immunol 2002; 168:4772–4780.
40. Pitti RM, Marsters SA, Lawrence DA, et al. Genomic amplification of a decoy receptor for Fas ligand in lung and colon cancer. Nature 1998; 396:699–703.
41. Roth W, Isenmann S, Nakamura M, et al. Soluble decoy receptor 3 is expressed by malignant gliomas and suppresses CD95 ligand-induced apoptosis and chemotaxis. Cancer Res 2001; 61:2759–2765.
42. Yu JS, Wheeler CJ, Zeltzer PM, et al. Vaccination of malignant glioma patients with peptide-pulsed dendritic cells elicits systemic cytotoxicity and intracranial T-cell infiltration. Cancer Res 2001; 61:842–847.
43. Yu JS, Liu G, Ying H, et al. Vaccination with tumor lysate-pulsed dendritic cells elicits antigen-specific, cytotoxic T-cells in patients with malignant glioma. Cancer Res 2004; 64:4973–4979.
44. Kikuchi T, Akasaki Y, Irie M, et al. Results of a phase I clinical trial of vaccination of glioma patients with fusions of dendritic and glioma cells. Cancer Immunol Immunother 2001; 50:337–344.
45. Kikuchi T, Akasaki Y, Abe T, et al. Vaccination of glioma patients with fusions of dendritic and glioma cells and recombinant human interleukin 12. J Immunother (1997) 2004; 27:452–459.
46. Akasaki Y, Kikuchi T, Homma S, et al. Antitumor effect of immunizations with fusions of dendritic and glioma cells in a mouse brain tumor model. J Immunother 2001; 24:106–113.

47. Akasaki Y, Black KL, Yu JS. Dendritic cell-based immunotherapy for malignant gliomas. Expert Rev Neurother 2005; 5:497–508.
48. Ehtesham M, Kabos P, Gutierrez MA, et al. Intratumoral dendritic cell vaccination elicits potent tumoricidal immunity against malignant glioma in rats. J Immunother 2003; 26:107–116.
49. Yamanaka R, Abe T, Yajima N, et al. Vaccination of recurrent glioma patients with tumour lysate-pulsed dendritic cells elicits immune responses: results of a clinical phase I/II trial. Br J Cancer 2003; 89:1172–1179.
50. Inaba K, Inaba M, Naito M, et al. Dendritic cell progenitors phagocytose particulates, including bacillus Calmette–Guérin organisms, and sensitize mice to mycobacterial antigens in vivo. J Exp Med 1993; 178:479–488.
51. Yamanaka R, Homma J, Yajima N, et al. Clinical evaluation of dendritic cell vaccination for patients with recurrent glioma: results of a clinical phase I/II trial. Clin Cancer Res 2005; 11:4160–4167.
52. Liau LM, Prins RM, Kiertscher SM, et al. Dendritic cell vaccination in glioblastoma patients induces systemic and intracranial T-cell responses modulated by the local central nervous system tumor microenvironment. Clin Cancer Res 2005; 11:5515–5525.
53. Bredel M, Zentner J. Brain-tumour drug resistance: the bare essentials. Lancet Oncol 2002; 3:397–406.
54. Wakahara Y, Nawa A, Okamoto T, et al. Combination effect of anti-Fas antibody and chemotherapeutic drugs in ovarian cancer cells in vitro. Oncology 1997; 54:48–54.
55. Shtil AA, Turner JG, Durfee J, et al. Cytokine-based tumor cell vaccine is equally effective against parental and isogenic multidrug-resistant myeloma cells: the role of cytotoxic T lymphocytes. Blood 1999; 93:1831–1837.
56. Melguizo C, Prados J, Marchal JA, et al. Modulation of HLA class I expression in multidrug-resistant human rhabdomyosarcoma cells. Neoplasma 2003; 50:91–96.
57. Fisk B, Ioannides CG. Increased sensitivity of adriamycin-selected tumor lines to CTL-mediated lysis results in enhanced drug sensitivity. Cancer Res 1998; 58:4790–4793.
58. Pich A, Rancourt C. A role for intracellular immunization in chemosensitization of tumor cells? Gene Ther 1999; 6:1202–1209.
59. Liu G, Akasaki Y, Khong HT, et al. Cytotoxic T cell targeting of TRP-2 sensitizes human malignant glioma to chemotherapy. Oncogene 2005; 24:5226–5234.
60. Liu G, Khong HT, Wheeler CJ, et al. Molecular and functional analysis of tyrosinase-related protein (TRP)-2 as a cytotoxic T lymphocyte target in patients with malignant glioma. J Immunother 2003; 26:301–312.
61. Bauman GS, Ino Y, Ueki K, et al. Allelic loss of chromosome 1p and radiotherapy plus chemotherapy in patients with oligodendrogliomas. Int J Radiat Oncol Biol Phys 2000; 48:825–830.
62. Cairncross JG, Ueki K, Zlatescu MC, et al. Specific genetic predictors of chemotherapeutic response and survival in patients with anaplastic oligodendrogliomas. J Natl Cancer Inst 1998; 90:1473–1479.
63. Newsham IF, Gorse KM, Rempel SA, et al. Use of horizontal ultrathin gel electrophoresis to analyze allelic deletions in chromosome band 11p15.5 in gliomas. Neurooncol 2000; 2:1–5.
64. Wheeler CJ, Black KL. Dendritic cell vaccines and immunity in glioma patients. Front Biosci 2005; 10:2861–2881.
65. Khong HT, Restifo NP. Natural selection of tumor variants in the generation of "tumor escape" phenotypes. Nat Immunol 2002; 3:999–1005.

66. Dunn GP, Bruce AT, Ikeda H, et al. Cancer immunoediting: from immuno-surveillance to tumor escape. Nat Immunol 2002; 3:991–998.

67. Nair S, Boczkowski D, Moeller B, et al. Synergy between tumor immunotherapy and antiangiogenic therapy. Blood 2003; 102:964–971.

68. Liu G, Ying H, Zeng G, et al. HER-2, gp100, and MAGE-1 are expressed in human glioblastoma and recognized by cytotoxic T cells. Cancer Res 2004; 64:4980–4986.

69. Nowak AK, Robinson BW, Lake RA. Synergy between chemotherapy and immu-notherapy in the treatment of established murine solid tumors. Cancer Res 2003; 63:4490–4496.

70. Gribben JG, Ryan DP, Boyajian R, et al. Unexpected association between induction of immunity to the universal tumor antigen CYP1B1 and response to next therapy. Clin Cancer Res 2005; 11:4430–4436.

71. Liu G, Black KL, Yu JS. Sensitization of malignant glioma to chemotherapy through dendritic cell vaccination. Expert Rev Vaccines 2006; 5:233–247.

72. Ehtesham M, Yuan X, Kabos P, et al. Glioma tropic neural stem cells consist of astrocytic precursors and their migratory capacity is mediated by CXCR4. Neoplasia 2004; 6:287–293.

73. Yuan X, Curtin J, Xiong Y, et al. Isolation of cancer stem cells from adult glio-blastoma multiforme. Oncogene 2004; 23:9392–9400.

74. Singh SK, Hawkins C, Clarke ID, et al. Identification of human brain tumour initiating cells. Nature 2004; 432:396–401.

75. Singh SK, Clarke ID, Terasaki M, et al. Identification of a cancer stem cell in human brain tumors. Cancer Res 2003; 63:5821–5828.

76. Hemmati HD, Nakano I, Lazareff JA, et al. Cancerous stem cells can arise from pediatric brain tumors. Proc Natl Acad Sci USA 2003; 100:15178–15183.

77. Salmaggi A, Boiardi A, Gelati M, et al. Glioblastoma-derived tumorospheres identify a population of tumor stem-like cells with angiogenic potential and enhanced mul-tidrug resistance phenotype. Glia 2006; 54:850–860.

78. Liu G, Yuan X, Zeng Z, et al. Analysis of gene expression and chemoresistance of CD133+ cancer stem cells in glioblastoma. Mol Cancer 2006; 5:67.

79. Bao S, Wu Q, McLendon RE, et al. Glioma stem cells promote radioresistance by preferential activation of the DNA damage response. Nature 2006; 444:756–760.

80. Pellegatta S, Poliani PL, Corno D, et al. Neurospheres enriched in cancer stem-like cells are highly effective in eliciting a dendritic cell-mediated immune response against malignant gliomas. Cancer Res 2006; 66:10247–10252.

81. Tunici P, Irvin D, Liu G, et al. Brain tumor stem cells: new targets for clinical treatments? Neurosurg Focus 2006; 20:E27.

82. Lake RA, Robinson BW. Immunotherapy and chemotherapy: a practical partnership. Nat Rev Cancer 2005; 5:397–405.

83. Emens LA, Jaffee EM. Leveraging the activity of tumor vaccines with cytotoxic chemotherapy. Cancer Res 2005; 65:8059–8064.

84. Zou W. Immunosuppressive networks in the tumour environment and their thera-peutic relevance. Nat Rev Cancer 2005; 5:263–274.

85. Akasaki Y, Liu G, Chung NH, et al. Induction of a CD4+ T regulatory type 1 response by cyclooxygenase-2-overexpressing glioma. J Immunol 2004; 173:4352–4359.

86. Rosenberg SA, Yang JC, Restifo NP. Cancer immunotherapy: moving beyond current vaccines. Nat Med 2004; 10:909–915.

6

Peptide-Based Active Immunotherapy in Cancer

Stephanie Schroter

*Laboratory of Genetics, Salk Institute for Biological Sciences,
La Jolla, California, U.S.A.*

Boris Minev

*Rebecca and John Moores UCSD Cancer Center,
La Jolla, California, U.S.A.*

INTRODUCTION

Cancer vaccines exemplify active specific immunotherapy—i.e., specific stimulation of patient's immune system against cancer. Improved understanding of the molecular mechanisms of antigen processing and presentation and the identification of tumor-associated antigens (TAA) in melanoma and other cancers have allowed the development of specific vaccines. T lymphocytes recognize tumor antigenic epitopes—peptides bound to the MHC molecules. Importantly, these peptide epitopes allow for precise direction of the antitumor immune responses.

Class II MHC molecules present peptides of 12–25 amino acids, with a groove-contacting region in the middle and side chains of several amino acids (1). Class II-binding peptides are generally of extracellular origin and are predominantly recognized by CD4+ T lymphocytes (2). The cytotoxic T lymphocytes (CTL) expressing CD8 molecules recognize class I-restricted peptides, mostly of 8–10 residues, which are the products of intracellularly processed proteins (2,3). Cytosolic peptides are transported across the endoplasmic reticulum (ER) membrane with the help of the ATP-dependent transporters associated with antigen processing (TAP) (4,5). Peptides complexed with class I molecules in the ER are then transported to the cell surface for recognition by CTL (3,6). The interaction between CTL and the target tumor cells begins with the binding of the peptide antigen associated with the MHC class I molecule to the T-cell antigen receptor. Lymphocyte-mediated cytolysis is further enhanced by accessory molecules, such as lymphocyte function antigen-1 and -3, costimulatory molecules (CD28, B7), and the intercellular adhesion molecule-1 (7), among others.

The realization that MHC class I–restricted tumor antigens can act as targets for CTL (8) promoted the search for tumor antigen genes (9,10). CTL appear to be among the most direct and effective elements of the immune system that are capable of generating antitumor immune responses (11). Tumor cells expressing the appropriate TAA can be effectively recognized and destroyed by these immune effector cells, which may result in dramatic clinical responses (12–14). Both the adoptive transfer of tumor-reactive CTL and active immunization designed to elicit CTL responses have been reported to lead to significant therapeutic antitumor responses in some patients (12–14). However, currently there are no human peptide–based vaccines on the market—resulting primarily from difficulties associated with peptide stability and delivery, and the diversity of human target antigens. Therefore, further research aimed at enhancing the stability and immunogenicity of the peptides used for vaccination of patients with cancer is essential.

TUMOR-ASSOCIATED ANTIGENS

Identification of highly expressed TAA is essential to the development of potent and specific cancer vaccines. A variety of approaches have been used for the identification of TAA recognized by CTL, including screening cDNA expression libraries with tumor-reactive CTL (11), testing of known proteins for recognition by CTL (15), direct isolation and sequencing of peptides eluted from the tumor cells (16,17), and serological analysis of recombinant cDNA expression libraries of human tumors with autologous serum (SEREX) (18). More recently, computer programs have been used to identify peptide sequences of known proteins based on their binding affinity for selected HLA molecules. We analyzed the sequence of human telomerase reverse transcriptase (hTRT) for peptide sequences binding to the HLA-A2.1 molecule and demonstrated that the hTRT peptide-specific CTL of normal individuals and patients with cancer specifically lysed a variety of HLA-A2+ cancer cell lines (19). Using different computer-based algorithms, we identified six epitopes recognized by human CTL within the sequence of the new tumor-associated antigen MG50 (20).

Utilizing these approaches, many melanoma target antigens and antigen-derived peptides have been identified, including tyrosinase, MART-1/Melan-A, gp100, TRP1/gp75, TRP2, MAGE, BAGE, GAGE, RAGE, NY-ESO-1, and others (11,21). In breast cancer and other adenocarcinomas, a polymorphic epithelial mucin (22) and HER2/neu proto-oncogene (23) have been characterized as tumor antigens.

Promising novel approaches for identification of TAA have been developed recently. Applying a combination of techniques, such as "suppression subtractive hybridization" and "transmembrane trapping," Di Cristina et al. identified a large panel of cDNA fragments encoding a variety of TAA, representing novel tumor-specific targets (24). Furukawa et al. studied the roles of ganglioside GD3 in human malignant melanomas and those of GD2 in small cell lung cancer as modulators of the malignant properties of cancer, suggesting their function as novel targets for cancer therapy (25). Recently, it was found that regulator of G-protein signaling 5 (RGS5) is broadly unregulated in a wide variety of malignant cells and that RGS5-specific CTL lines possess antigen-specific and HLA-restricted cytolytic activity against tumor cells (26). Newly identified TAA-derived peptides also demonstrated a strong potential to be particularly useful in the treatment of hematologic malignancies (27,28).

In contrast to class I TAA, little attention has been paid to the identification of class II TAA, mostly because of the difficulties in their identification. However, a growing number of studies confirm the important role of CD4+ T cells in controlling tumor growth (29). Several important studies on cancer patients demonstrated the essential role of the CD4+ T cells for optimal CTL induction (30,31). Klyushnenkova et al. were able to successfully stimulate CD4+ T lymphocytes from HLA-DRB1*1501-positive donors, with prostatic acid phosphatase–derived class II–restricted peptides showing their potential as a new target for peptide-based immunotherapy (32). These findings confirm that tumor-specific CD4+ T lymphocytes are required for optimal induction of CTL against the autologous tumors. Therefore, both class I and class II peptides should be used to optimize the therapeutic effect of the peptide-based cancer vaccines.

PRECLINICAL AND CLINICAL STUDIES

The identification of peptide sequences recognized by CTL has led to attempts to directly induce CTL responses in vivo (33,34). Successful immunization of mice has been accomplished with peptides formulated with immunostimulating complex (35), entrapped in liposomes (36), encapsulated in microspheres (37), and osmotically loaded into syngeneic splenocytes (38) or coated on their surface (39). Effective immune responses were also elicited in mice with a mutant p53 peptide in adjuvant (40), or with either mutant or wild-type p53 peptides loaded on dendritic cells (41). We showed in two murine antigenic systems that fusion peptides with a synthetic ER signal sequence at the NH_2-terminus of the minimal peptide were more effective than the minimal peptide alone in generating specific CTL responses (42). Furthermore, we found that the CTL response was MHC class II independent, could not be attributed to increased hydrophobicity of the fusion peptides, and was very effective in prolonging the survival of tumor-challenged mice. More recently, we identified two HLA-A2.1-restricted peptides from hTRT and demonstrated that in vivo immunization of HLA-A2.1 transgenic mice generated a specific CTL response against both hTRT peptides (19). Based on the induction of CTL responses in vitro and in vivo, and the susceptibility to lysis of tumor cells of various origins by hTRT-specific CTL, we suggested that hTRT could serve as a universal cancer vaccine. Recently, Adotevi et al. identified CTL epitopes in hTRT restricted by HLA-B*0702 molecule, a common MHC class I allele (43). These new epitopes were found to induce primary human CTL against various hTRT-positive tumor cells. To study the clinical application of hTRT, Brunsvig et al. conducted a phase I/II study in patients will non-small cell lung cancer (NSCLC) (44). The authors investigated the safety, tolerability, and clinical response to vaccination with a combination of telomerase-derived peptides. Twenty-six patients received intradermal (i.d.) administrations of these peptides and granulocyte-macro-phage colony-stimulating factor (GM-CSF). It was found that the treatment was well tolerated with minor side effects and the selected peptides are immunogenic and safe to use in patients with NSCLC.

Increasing number of studies report peptide vaccination of cancer patients (Table 1). Spontaneous CTL reactivity against the melanoma antigens Melan A/ MART-1, tyrosinase, and gp100 is frequently detected in melanoma patients and healthy individuals (45–47). These findings suggest that CTL responses against "self" antigens are induced spontaneously in patients and healthy individuals and may be boosted by appropriate vaccination. Immunizations with a MAGE-3-derived peptide without any adjuvant induced limited tumor regressions in five out of 17 patients with melanoma (48). More recently, the same group used an HLA-A1-restricted MAGE-3 peptide to immunize 39 patients with metastatic melanoma. Of the 25 patients who received the complete treatment, seven displayed significant tumor regressions: three regressions were complete and two led to a disease-free state, which persisted for more than two years after the beginning of treatment (49). Salgaller et al. reported generation of CTL specific for one of three gp100-derived peptides in patients vaccinated with peptide in incomplete Freund's adjuvant (IFA) (50). Immunization of three patients with advanced melanoma with peptide-pulsed autologous antigen-presenting cells led to induction of peptide-specific CTL (51). The peptide used in this study was derived from MAGE-1 and was restricted to HLA-A1.1. The lack of any therapeutic response observed in this trial might be explained by the advanced stage of the disease in these patients. In another study, nine melanoma patients were vaccinated weekly for four weeks with a combination of peptides derived from MART-1, tyrosinase, and gp100 proteins (52). Successful immunization against peptides could be detected in vitro in two of six patients against the tyrosinase peptide, three of six patients against the MART-1 peptide, and none of six patients receiving the gp100 peptide. More recently, 18 patients with melanoma were immunized with a peptide derived from MART-1, emulsified with IFA (34). An enhancement of cytotoxic activity against MART-1 was detected with minimal toxicity for patients with local irritation at the site of

(text continues on page 117)

Table 1 Investigational Peptide-Based Vaccines

Antigen	Tumor type	Strategy	Development stage	Biological/clinical activity	Reference
Alpha-fetoprotein	Liver cancer	Monotherapy	Phase I	All of the six patients' T-cell repertoire was capable of recognizing alpha-fetoprotein as determined by ELISPOT and MHC Class I tetramer assays	81
gp100	Melanoma	Monotherapy	Phase II	No objective tumor responses or severe toxicities. Four patients remained progression free for over 100 days. Ten of 21 patients had an increased frequency of vaccine-specific, nonfunctional cytotoxic T lymphocytes.	55
gp100	Melanoma	Monotherapy	Phase I/II	CTL responses in 91% of patients. Clinical responses in 42% of patients receiving the peptide vaccine plus IL-2	13
gp100	Melanoma	Combinatorial (anti-CTLA-4 antibody)	Phase I/II	Two complete responses and one partial response in 14 patients with stage IV melanoma that were maintained beyond 12 mo	63
gp100	Melanoma	Monotherapy	Phase I	In vitro detection of successful immunization in 0 of 6 patients	52
gp100, MART-1/Melan-A, tyrosinase	Melanoma	Combinatorial (anti-CTLA-4 antibody)	Phase I	Nine of 11 patients without autoimmune symptoms had disease relapse, and 3 of 8 patients with autoimmune symptoms had relapse	64
gp100 and tyrosinase	Melanoma	Combinatorial (tetanus helper peptide and IL-2)	Phase II	Twenty out of 40 vaccinated patients had T-cell responses by ELISPOT. Disease-free survival was 50% for the gp100 group and 39% for the tyrosinase group at 2 yr	75

Table 1 Investigational Peptide-Based Vaccines (*Continued*)

Antigen	Tumor type	Strategy	Development stage	Biological/clinical activity	Reference
gp100 and tyrosinase	Melanoma	Combinatorial (IL-12)	Phase I	Thirty-four out of 40 patients developed a positive skin test response to only the gp100 peptide and not the tyrosinase peptide. Thirty-three out of 38 patients had an immune response by ELISA, and 37 out of 42 patients had an immune response by tetramer assay	76
HER-2/neu	Prostate cancer	Combinatorial (flt3 ligand)	Phase I	No significant peptide-specific T-cell responses were detected	83
HER-2/neu	Breast cancer	Combinatorial (GM-CSF)	Phase I	CD4+ T cell recruitment and a significant decrease in circulating regulatory T cells and TGF-beta levels	84, 85
hTRT	Breast and prostate cancer	Monotherapy	Phase I	hTRT-specific T lymphocytes were induced in 4 of 7 patients; no significant toxicity	82
hTRT	non-small cell lung cancer	Combinatorial (GM-CSF)	Phase I/II	Peptides were found safe and immunogenic in all 26 patients	44
MAGE-1	Melanoma	Monotherapy	Phase I	All vaccinated patients generated peptide-specific CTL. No therapeutic response was observed	51
MAGE-A1, MAGE-A10, and gp100	Melanoma	Combinatorial (GM-CSF)	Phase I	Peptide-specific T cells were detected in peripheral blood and in the sentinel immunized node	78
MAGE-3	Melanoma	Monotherapy	Phase I	Limited tumor regressions in five out of 17 patients	48
MAGE-3	Melanoma	Monotherapy	Phase I	Significant tumor regressions in 7 out of 25 patients	49
MART-1/Melan-A	Melanoma	Monotherapy	Phase I	In vitro detection of successful immunization in 3 of 6 patients	52

MART-1/Melan-A	Melanoma	Monotherapy	Phase I	No tumor regression observed. An enhancement of the cytotoxic activity against MART-1/Melan-A was detected	34
MART-1/Melan-A, gp100, and tyrosinase	Melanoma	Combinatorial (SD-9427—a GM-CSF agonist)	Phase I	Six of 12 patients developed a positive skin test response to the peptides. Seven of 10 patients had an immune response to at least one peptide when evaluated via IFN-gamma release assay and ELISPOT assay, so did 11 of 12 patients analyzed by MHC-peptide tetramer assay	80
MART-1/Melan-A	Melanoma	Monotherapy	Phase I	Ten of 22 patients had response to peptide-pulsed targets or tumor cells by ELISA assay after vaccination. Twelve of 20 patients had response by ELISPOT. Immune response by ELISA correlated with prolonged relapse-free survival	65
MART-1/Melan-A	Melanoma	Combinatorial (IL-12)	Phase II	Out of 20 patients, two patients had a complete response, five had a minor or mixed response, and four patients had stable disease. There was a correlation between the magnitude of the increase in MART-1/Melan-A-specific cells and clinical response	77
MART-1/Melan-A, tyrosinase, MAGE-3	Melanoma	Combinatorial (Montanide-ISA-720 adjuvant, GM-CSF)	Phase I/II	Peptides were more effective when given with the adjuvant Montanide-ISA-720	79

(Continued)

Table 1 Investigational Peptide-Based Vaccines (*Continued*)

Antigen	Tumor type	Strategy	Development stage	Biological/clinical activity	Reference
NY-ESO-1	Melanoma	Monotherapy	Phase I/II	Stabilization of disease and regression of individual metastases in 3 of 12 patients. Induction of CTL-specific responses	53
ras	Pancreatic cancer	Monotherapy	Phase I/II	Induction of cancer cell–specific cellular response. No side effects	54
SART, Lck, ART, PAP, PSA, PSMA, MRP	Prostate cancer	Combinatorial RRP was performed	Phase I/II	Vaccination was well tolerated. In 8 out of the 10 patients increased CTL response and anti-peptide IgG titer were observed. CD8+ T cell infiltration was increased at the tumor site	56
SART, Lck, ART, PAP, PSA, PSMA, MRP	Prostate cancer	Combinatorial (EMP)	Phase I/II	Well tolerated. In 27 of 37 patients, increased levels of CTL precursors were found; in 36 of 41 patients, increased IgG responses were observed	57
Tyrosinase	Melanoma	Monotherapy	Phase I	In vitro detection of successful immunization in 2 of 6 patients	52

Abbreviations: RRP, retropubic radical prostatectomy; EMP, estramustine phosphate.

vaccination. Serial administrations of this peptide appeared to boost the level of cytotoxicity in vitro, although clinical regression of the tumor was not observed. Peptides derived from NY-ESO-1, one of the most immunogenic tumor antigens, were used to immunize 12 patients with metastatic NY-ESO-1 expressing cancers, including melanoma (53). This trial demonstrated induction of primary NY-ESO-1-specific CTL responses as well as stabilization of disease and regression of individual metastases in three patients. In another trial, patients with advanced pancreatic carcinoma were vaccinated with a synthetic ras peptide pulsed on antigen-presenting cells isolated from peripheral blood (54). This procedure led to generation of cancer cell–specific cellular response, without side effects. However, in all patients, tumor progression was observed after the vaccination. Based on promising preclinical results, Celis et al. conducted a clinical trial using the MPS160 vaccine in patients with metastatic melanoma. MPS160 is a gp 100–derived melanoma peptide that contains overlapping HLA-A2–, DR53-, and DQw6-restricted T-cell epitopes. It was found that none of the 28 patients exhibited objective tumor responses or severe toxicities, and that four of the 28 patients remained progression free for over 100 days. Based on immunologic analysis for 21 patients, it was determined that vaccination increased the frequency of vaccine-specific, nonfunctional CTL in 10 patients, and there was evidence of systemic cytokine/immune dysfunction (55). Noguchi et al. recently performed two well-designed clinical trials with prostate cancer patients. In the first trial the safety and immune responses to a personalized peptide vaccine were evaluated in preoperative prostate cancer (56). Ten HLA-A24+ patients with localized prostate cancer received the peptide vaccine weekly, and soon after vaccination, a retropubic radical prostatectomy was performed. It was found that the peptide vaccination was safe and well tolerated with no major side effects. In eight out of the 10 patients, increased CTL response and anti-peptide IgG titer was observed. CD8+ T cell infiltration was also increased at the tumor site. In the second study, the prognostic factors of patients with metastatic hormone refractory prostate cancer (HRPC) were studied. Fifty-eight patients with metastatic HRPC received a combination therapy of personalized peptide vaccination and low-dose estramustine phosphate (57). Results showed that there were no major side effects and that this vaccine was also well tolerated. In 27 of 37 patients, increased levels of CTL precursors were found, and in 36 of 41 patients, increased IgG responses were observed. Also, a prostate-specific antigen decline of at least 50% occurred in 24% of patients.

OPTIMIZING PEPTIDE-BASED VACCINES

Several strategies for modifying peptides have been attempted to improve their efficiency as cancer vaccines. The clinical use of peptides is limited by their rapid proteolytic digestion. To overcome this limitation, Celis et al. designed a peptide construct containing a pan-reactive DR epitope, a CTL epitope, and a fatty-acid moiety (58). A lipopeptide-based therapeutic vaccine was able to induce strong CTL responses both in humans and in animals (59). Several studies demonstrated a correlation between MHC binding affinity and peptide immunogenicity (60). Peptides derived from gp100, whose anchor residues were modified to fit the optimal HLA-A2 binding motif, stimulated tumor-reactive CTL more efficiently than the natural epitopes (61). An unmodified, gp100-derived peptide failed to elicit peptide-specific CTL in melanoma patients after subcutaneous administration with IFA. In contrast, vaccination with the modified peptide induced CTL responses in 91% of cases (13). None of the 11 patients immunized with the modified peptide in IFA alone experienced an objective tumor response. Interestingly, administration of the modified peptide along with high-dose interleukin-2 (IL-2) led to a clinical response rate of 42% in a group of 31 patients. More recently, Eguchi et al. identified the IL-13 receptor alpha2 (IL-13Ralpha2) peptide as an HLA-A2-restricted CTL epitope (62). IL-13Ralpha2 is restricted to, and expressed at, high levels in a majority of human malignant gliomas, making this protein an attractive vaccine target. ThreeIL-13Ralpha2 analogue peptides were created by substitutions of amino acids at the COOH-terminal. Compared to the native IL-13Ralpha2 epitope, the analogue peptides displayed higher levels of binding affinity and stability in HLA-A2 complexes. They also yielded improved stimulation of patient-derived, specific CTL against the native epitope expressed by HLA-A2+ glioma cells. In transgenic mice, immunization with these two modified peptides induced enhanced levels of CTL reactivity and protective immunity against IL13Ralpha2-expressing syngeneic tumors when compared with vaccines containing the native IL-13Ralpha2 epitope (62). These findings illustrate the beneficial use of certain peptide modifications when developing optimized vaccines for cancer. Recently, two modified gp100 peptides were combined with an antibody that abrogated cytotoxic T lymphocyte antigen-4 (CTLA-4) signaling to augment T-cell reactivity (63). In that trial there were two complete responses and one partial response in 14 patients with stage IV melanoma that were maintained beyond 12 months. Another group also utilized the same anti-CTLA-4 antibody in combination with three melanoma peptides (64). Nineteen patients with stage III and IV melanoma were immunized. Nine of 11 patients without autoimmune symptoms have experienced disease relapse, and three of eight patients with autoimmune symptoms experienced relapse. These findings suggest possible correlation between development of autoimmunity and lack of relapse. Several groups reported clinical trials with melanoma patients immunized with the immunogenic peptide MART-1_{27-35} (AAGIGILTV) (65–67). Wang et al. immunized patients with high-risk resected melanoma with MART-1_{27-35} complexed with IFAs, or with Freund's adjuvants mixed with CRL1005, a blocked co-polymer adjuvant. Ten of 22 patients demonstrated an immune response to peptide-pulsed targets or tumor cells by ELISA assay after vaccination, as did 12 of 20 patients by ELISPOT. Immune response by ELISA correlated with prolonged relapse-free survival (65). These data suggest that a significant proportion of patients with resected melanoma mount an antigen-specific immune response against MART-1_{27-35}. Another study analyzed antigen-specific T-cell responses induced in the skin and in peripheral blood lymphocytes in a HLA-A2+ melanoma patient. The patient showed major regression of metastatic melanoma under continued immunization with peptides derived from the antigens MART-1, tyrosinase, and gp100 (66). The authors demonstrated that i.d. immunization with peptides alone leads to oligoclonal expansion of MART-1-specific CTL. These findings provide strong evidence for the effective induction of specific T-cell responses to MART-1 by i.d. immunization with peptide alone, which accounts for specific cytotoxicity against MART-1-expressing melanoma cells and clinical tumor regression. Brinckerhoff et al. evaluated the stability of the same peptide— MART-1$_{27-35}$—in fresh normal human plasma and possible peptide modifications that convey protection against enzymatic destruction without loss of immunogenicity (67). When this peptide was incubated in plasma prior to pulsing on target cells, CTL reactivity was lost within three hours. The stability of MART-1$_{27-35}$ was markedly prolonged by C-terminal amidation and/or N-terminal acetylation, or by polyethylene-glycol modification of the C-terminus. These modified peptides were recognized by CTL. This study suggests that the immunogenicity of the peptide vaccines might be enhanced by creating modifications that increase their stability.

We investigated the effectiveness of several synthetic insertion signal sequences in enhancing the presentation of the HLA-A2.1-restricted melanoma epitope MART-1$_{27-35}$ (68). An important step in presentation of the class I-restricted antigens is the translocation of processed proteins from the cytosol across the ER membrane mediated by TAP proteins, or as an alternative, by ER-insertion signal sequences located at the NH$_2$-terminus of the precursor molecules (69). Using a technique known as osmotic lysis of pinocytic vesicles (70), we loaded several synthetic peptide constructs into the cytosol of antigen processing deficient T2 cells, TAP-expressing human melanoma cells, and dendritic cells. We examined whether the natural signal sequences ES (derived from the adenovirus E3/19K glycoprotein) (71) and IS (derived from IFN-b) (72) could enhance and prolong presentation of MART-1$_{27-35}$. We found that the addition of signal sequence at the N-terminus, but not at the C-terminus, of MART-1$_{27-35}$ greatly enhanced its presentation in both TAP-deficient and TAP-expressing cells. A newly designed peptide construct, composed of the epitope replacing the hydrophobic part of a natural signal sequence, was also effective. Interestingly, an artificial signal sequence containing the epitope was the most efficient construct for enhancing its presentation. These peptide constructs facilitated epitope presentation in a TAP-independent manner when loaded into the cytosol of TAP-deficient T2 cells. In addition, loading of these constructs into TAP-expressing melanoma cells also led to a more efficient presentation than loading of the minimal peptide. Most importantly, loading of human dendritic cells with the same constructs resulted in a prolonged presentation of this melanoma epitope (68). The efficient presentation of MART-1$_{27-35}$, loaded into TAP-expressing tumor cells and dendritic cells, may be explained by the availability of intact TAP transporters in these cells. In this case, some of the loaded MART-1$_{27-35}$ may have been translocated by TAP from the cytosol even eight days after loading. The size of MART-1$_{27-35}$ (nine amino acids) is appropriate for optimal translocation by TAP (73). Still, fusion peptides were more effective than MART-1$_{27-35}$, probably because of their translocation by both TAP-dependent and TAP-independent pathways. The latter mechanism of peptide translocation may be important for antigen presentation especially in cancers that fail to utilize the classical MHC class I pathway (74). These findings may be of practical significance for the development of synthetic anticancer vaccines and in vitro immunization of CTL for adoptive immunotherapy.

Various methods have been exploited to improve the peptide vaccine antigenicity. The most common are a combination of the peptide administered with cytokines and/or with an adjuvant. Slingluff et al. implemented a phase II trial to test whether low-dose IL-2 is capable of enhancing T-cell immune responses to a multipeptide melanoma vaccine (75). Forty melanoma patients were randomly vaccinated with four gp100- and tyrosinase-derived peptides that were restricted by HLA-A1, -A2, and -A3. After either one week or 28 days, a tetanus helper peptide as well as IL-2 was administered daily. A higher response was found in the second group (tetanus helper peptide and IL-2 administered after 28 days). This study also found that the tyrosinase peptides DAEKS-DICTDEY and YMDGTMSQV were more immunogenic than the gp100 peptides YLEPGPVTA and ALLAVGATK. The disease-free survival estimates were 39% for the first group and 50% for the second group at two years. In another trial, the effect of IL-12 on the immune response to a resected metastatic melanoma multipeptide vaccine was studied in 48 patients with melanoma (76). The patients were immunized with two peptides derived from gp100(209–217 (210M)) and tyrosinase(368–376 (370D)) emulsified with IFA. The peptide/adjuvant was either administered with or without IL-12. Out of 40 patients, 34 developed a positive skin test response to only the gp100 peptide and not the tyrosinase peptide. Out of 38 patients, 33 showed an immune response as determined by ELISA, and 37 of 42 patients showed a response by a tetramer assay. These findings indicate that IL-12 may augment the immune response to certain peptides. These findings were confirmed by Peterson et al. who found in a phase II study that recombinant IL-12 when administered with MART-1/Melan-A is effective as an adjuvant in melanoma patients (77). Another recent trial determined that the melanoma peptides MAGE-A1 (96–104), MAGE-A10 (254–262), and gp100(614–622) are immunogenic when combined with GM-CSF and montanide-ISA-51 adjuvant and administered as part of a multipeptide vaccine (78). Hersey et al. undertook a phase I/II trial with 36 patients with melanoma, half of whom were given peptides derived from gp100, MART-1, tyrosinase, and MAGE-3 in the Montanide-ISA-720 adjuvant, and half the patients were given GM-CSF subcutaneously for four days following each injection (79). The authors concluded that the peptides were more effective when given with the adjuvant Montanide-ISA-720. In another trial the peptides MART-1(26–35 (27L)), gp100(209–217 (210M)), and tyrosinase(368–376 (370D)) were emulsified with IFA and administered with SD-9427 (progenipoietin)—an agonist of granulocyte colony-stimulating factor and the FLT-3 receptor (80). This study found that the SD-9427 combined with a multipeptide vaccine was generally well tolerated, and that the majority of patients with resected melanoma mounted an antigen-specific immune response against the multipeptide vaccine. Butterfield et al. studied the induction of T-cell responses to HLA-A*0201 immunodominant peptides derived from alpha-fetoprotein (AFP) in patients with hepatocellular cancer (81). In this study the authors tested the immunologic paradigm that high concentrations of soluble protein contribute to the maintenance of peripheral tolerance/ignorance to self-protein. They confirmed that the patients' T-cell repertoire was capable of recognizing AFP in the context of MHC class I even in an environment of high circulating levels of this oncofetal protein. Our group identified two HLA-A2-restricted peptides derived from hTRT, and induced hTRT-specific CTL in vitro (19). More important, we also demonstrated that the hTRT-specific CTL lysed a variety of HLA-A2-positive cancer cell lines, but not HLA-A2-negative cancer cell lines. All of these cancer cell lines were hTRT positive as determined by the TRAPeze assay (Intergen). A phase I clinical trial was performed by Vonderheide et al. to evaluate the clinical and immunologic impact of vaccinating advanced cancer patients with the HLA-A2-restricted hTRT I540 peptide presented with keyhole limpet hemocyanin by ex vivo generated autologous dendritic cells (82). It was found that hTRT-specific T lymphocytes were induced in four of seven patients with advanced breast or prostate carcinoma after vaccination with dendritic cells pulsed with hTRT peptide. It is important to note that no significant toxicity was observed despite concerns of telomerase activity in rare normal cells. These results demonstrated the immunologic feasibility of vaccinating patients against telomerase and provided rationale for targeting self-antigens with critical roles in oncogenesis. An interesting study utilized the flt3 ligand as a systemic vaccine adjuvant with the E75 HLA-A2 epitope from HER-2/neu (83). Twenty patients with advanced-stage prostate cancer were enrolled in this study. Dendritic cells were markedly increased in the peripheral blood of subjects receiving flt3 ligand with each repetitive cycle, but augmentation of antigen-presenting cells within the dermis was not observed. No significant peptide-specific T-cell responses were detected. The authors concluded that the inability of fit3 ligand to augment the number of peripheral skin antigen-presenting cells may have contributed to the absence of robust peptide-specific immunity detectable in the peripheral blood of immunized subjects treated with flt3 ligand. Recently, Hueman et al. performed clinical trials in breast cancer patients to test the HER2/neu peptide vaccine (E75) (84,85). Blood samples from 22 healthy individuals and 22 patients, including pre- and post-vaccination samples from seven vaccinated HLA-A2+ patients, were obtained. Vaccination with E75 resulted in CD4+ T cell recruitment and was associated with a significant decrease in circulating regulatory T cells and TGF-beta levels in the majority of the vaccinated patients. These results illustrate that successful cancer vaccination strategies may require the modification of complex immune interactions.

CONSIDERATIONS ON PEPTIDE VACCINE DESIGN AND APPLICATION

A difficulty with the use of peptide vaccines is the fact that the T-cell responses usually do not last long enough to have a significant effect on the tumor. To address this issue, Davila et al. examined the role of synthetic oligodeoxynucleotide (ODN) adjuvants containing unmethylated cytosine-guanine motifs (CpG-ODN) and CTLA-4 blockade in enhancing the antitumor effectiveness of peptide vaccines intended to elicit CTL responses (86). This study found that combination immunotherapy consisting of vaccination with a synthetic peptide corresponding to an immunodominant CTL epitope derived from tyrosinase-related protein-2 administered with CpG-ODN adjuvant and followed by systemic injection of anti-CTLA-4 antibodies increased the survival of mice against the poorly immunogenic B16 melanoma. These findings suggest that peptide vaccination applied in combination with a strong adjuvant and CTLA-4 blockade is capable of eliciting durable antitumor T-cell responses that provide survival benefit. These findings bear clinical significance for the design of peptide-based therapeutic vaccines for cancer patients.

From a clinical perspective, immunization with peptides may be preferable to immunization with recombinant vaccinia viruses because of its safety and because it is not associated with diminished immune responses in patients immunized against smallpox. Immunizing with minimal determinant constructs may avoid the possible oncogenic effect of full-length proteins containing ras, p53, or other potential oncogenes. In addition to their safety, peptide vaccines can be designed to induce well-defined immune responses and synthesized in large quantities with very high purity and reproducibility. Another potential advantage of peptide vaccines over whole proteins or DNA vaccines is the ability to identify the specific epitopes of the tumor antigens to which an individual is able to mount an immune response, but not a state of immune tolerance (87). In addition, in vivo or in vitro immunization with peptide antigens "packaged" in dendritic cells or other antigen-presenting cells (discussed below) opens an exciting opportunity for eliciting powerful CTL responses.

A disadvantage of peptide vaccines is their poor immunogenicity and monospecificity of the induced immune response. Another limiting factor for the use of peptide vaccines in outbred populations is that T cells from individuals expressing different MHC molecules recognize different peptides from tumor or viral antigens in the context of self-MHC. However, the use of synthetic peptides from TAA that are presented by common MHC molecules may overcome this problem. Poor immunogenicity caused by rapid degradation of the peptides by serum peptidases may be corrected by modifications or incorporation of the peptides into controlled release formulations. Overall, personalized peptide vaccines may serve as an efficient therapeutic modality for cancer (88).

PROSPECTS

The growing number of TAA identified in many tumor types becomes a solid basis for peptide vaccine development. However, the antigenic profile of human tumors is very complex and consists of many peptides originating from various classes of protein. This fact should be considered carefully in designing anticancer vaccines. An important question is which tumor antigens are the most important in tumor regression in vivo. In any case, the ideal peptide vaccine most likely will consist of a cocktail of tumor antigenic peptides. However, the number of epitopes in the vaccine cocktail should be evaluated carefully since CTL responses in AIDS patients directed to fewer epitopes are associated with better clinical outcome (89). In this case it appears that the stimulation of multiple simultaneous CTL responses is clinically inefficient. The dose of antigen and the speed of antigen release in the vaccine formulations are also very important. High doses of antigen released faster may induce T-cell tolerance (90). Immune tolerance may be due to fast expansion and subsequent elimination of specific T-cell clones, or to apoptosis induced by repeated stimulation of already stimulated T-cells in cell cycle (91,92). Therefore, it is essential to select as immunogens those epitopes against which tolerance has not been induced (93,94).

Currently, clinical responses to peptide vaccines, as determined by the criteria set for chemotherapy and radiation, have been difficult to assess. However, the lack of toxicity of peptide vaccines in patients with many different tumor types, and the clearly observed efficacy in some studies, support the use of peptide vaccination. Future peptide vaccine strategies will most likely focus on more potent and combined approaches for immunization. Applied in conjunction with surgery, radiotherapy, and/or chemotherapy, peptide vaccines can be effective in eliminating micro-metastases, in decreasing the immunosuppressive effects of the chemotherapy or radiotherapy, and in increasing the resistance to viral or bacterial infections frequently occurring in cancer patients. Recent advances in the design of polyvalent vaccines targeting several antigens are also very promising. In addition, the possibility to treat patients with peptide vaccines earlier in the course of the disease and to combine vaccines with other treatment modalities may also improve the vaccine efficacy. As a result, immunotherapy with peptide vaccines may become a major treatment modality of cancer in the near future.

REFERENCES

1. Rammensee HG, Friede T, Stevanoviic S. MHC ligands and peptide motifs: first listing. Immunogenetics 1995; 41:178–228.
2. Rammensee HG. Antigen presentation—recent developments. Int Arch Allergy Immunol 1996; 110:299–307.
3. Yewdell JW, Norbury CC, Bennink JR. Mechanisms of exogenous antigen presentation by MHC class I molecules in vitro and in vivo: implications for generating CD8+ T cell responses to infectious agents, tumors, transplants, and vaccines. Adv Immunol 1999; 73:1–77.

4. Heemels MT, Ploegh H. Generation, translocation, and presentation of MHC class I-restricted peptides. Annu Rev Biochem 1995; 64:463–491.

5. Spies T, Cerundolo V, Colonna M, et al. Presentation of viral antigen by MHC class I molecules is dependent on a putative peptide transporter heterodimer. Nature 1992; 355:644–646.

6. Lehner PJ, Cresswell P. Processing and delivery of peptides presented by MHC class I molecules. Curr Opin Immunol 1996; 8:59–67.

7. Liu CC, Young LH, Young JD. Lymphocyte-mediated cytolysis and disease. N Engl J Med 1996; 335:1651–1659.

8. Van Pel A, van der Bruggen P, Coulie PG, et al. Genes coding for tumor antigens recognized by cytolytic T lymphocytes. Immunol Rev 1995; 145:229–250.

9. De Plaen E, Lurquin C, Lethe B, et al. Identification of genes coding for tumor antigens recognized by cytolytic T lymphocytes. Methods 1997; 12:125–142.

10. Rosenberg SA. Cancer vaccines based on the identification of genes encoding cancer regression antigens. Immunol Today 1997; 18:175–182.

11. Wang RF. Human tumor antigens: implications for cancer vaccine development. J Mol Med 1999; 77(9):640–655.

12. Nestle FO, Alijagic S, Gilliet M, et al. Vaccination of melanoma patients with peptide- or tumor lysate-pulsed dendritic cells. Nat Med 1998; 4(3):328–332.

13. Rosenberg SA, Yang JC, Schwartzentruber DJ, et al. Immunologic and therapeutic evaluation of a synthetic peptide vaccine for the treatment of patients with metastatic melanoma. Nat Med 1998; 4(3):321–327.

14. Thurner B, Haendle I, Reoder C, et al. Vaccination with mage-3A1 peptide-pulsed mature, monocyte-derived dendritic cells expands specific cytotoxic T cells and induces regression of some metastases in advanced stage IV melanoma. J Exp Med 1999; 190(11):1669–1678.

15. Kawakami Y, Nishimura MI, Restifo NP, et al. T-cell recognition of human melanoma antigens. J Immunother 1993; 14:88–93.

16. Storkus WJ, Zeh HJD, Maeurer MJ, et al. Identification of human melanoma peptides recognized by class I restricted tumor infiltrating T lymphocytes. J Immunol 1993; 151:3719–3727.

17. Cox AL, Skipper J, Chen Y, et al. Identification of a peptide recognized by five melanoma-specific human cytotoxic T cell lines. Science 1994; 264:716–719.

18. Sahin U, Teureci O, Pfreundschuh M. Serological identification of human tumor antigens. Curr Opin Immunol 1997; 9(5):709–716.

19. Minev B, Hipp J, Firat H, et al. Cytotoxic T cell immunity against telomerase reverse transcriptase in humans. Proc Natl Acad Sci U S A 2000; 97(9):4796–4801.

20. Mitchell MS, Kan-Mitchell J, Minev BR, et al. A novel melanoma gene (MG50) encoding the interleukin 1 receptor antagonist and six epitopes recognized by human cytolytic T lymphocytes. Cancer Res 2000; 60(22):6448–6456.

21. Romero P, Cerottini JC, Speiser DE. The human T cell response to melanoma antigens. Adv Immunol 2006; 92:187–224.

22. Takahashi T, Makiguchi Y, Hinoda Y, et al. Expression of MUC1 on myeloma cells and induction of HLA-unrestricted CTL against MUC1 from a multiple myeloma patient. J Immunol 1994; 153:2102–2109.

23. Coussens L, Yang-Feng TL, Liao YC, et al. Tyrosine kinase receptor with extensive homology to EGF receptor shares chromosomal location with neu oncogene. Science 1985; 230:1132–1139.

24. Di Cristina M, Minenkova O, Pavoni E, et al. A novel approach for identification of tumor-associated antigens expressed on the surface of tumor cells. Int J Cancer 2006; 120:1293–1303.
25. Furukawa K, Hamamura K, Aixinjueluo W. Biosignals modulated by tumor-associated carbohydrate antigens: novel targets for cancer therapy. Ann N Y Acad Sci 2006; 1086:185–198.
26. Boss CN, Grunebach F, Brauer K, et al. Identification and characterization of T-cell epitopes deduced from RGS5, a novel broadly expressed tumor antigen. Clin Cancer Res 2007; 13(11):3347–3355.
27. Kawahara M, Hori T, Matsubara Y, et al. Identification of HLA class I-restricted tumor-associated antigens in adult T cell leukemia cells by mass spectrometric analysis. Exp Hematol 2006; 34(11):1496–1504.
28. Greiner J, Schmitt M, Li L, et al. Expression of tumor-associated antigens in acute myeloid leukemia: implications for specific immunotherapeutic approaches. Blood 2006; 108(13):4109–4117.
29. Toes REM, Ossendorp F, Offringa R, et al. CD4 T cells and their role in antitumor immune responses. J Exp Med 1999; 189(5):753–756.
30. Baxevanis CN, Voutsas IF, Tsitsilonis OE, et al. Tumor-specific CD4+ T lymphocytes from cancer patients are required for optimal induction of cytotoxic T cells against the autologous tumor. J Immunol 2000; 164(7):3902–3912.
31. Zarour HM, Kirkwood JM, Kierstead LS, et al. Melan-A/MART-1(51-73) represents an immunogenic HLA-DR4-restricted epitope recognized by melanoma-reactive CD4(+) T cells. Proc Natl Acad Sci U S A 2000; 97(1):400–405.
32. Klyushnenkova EN, Kouiavskaia DV, Kodak JA, et al. Identification of HLA-DRB1*1501-restricted T-cell epitopes from human prostatic acid phosphatase. Prostate 2007; 67(10):1019–1028.
33. Schulz M, Zinkernagel RM, Hengartner H. Peptide-induced antiviral protection by cytotoxic T cells. Proc Natl Acad Sci U S A 1991; 88:991–993.
34. Cormier JN, Salgaller ML, Prevette T, et al. Enhancement of cellular immunity in melanoma patients immunized with a peptide from MART-1/Melan A [see comments]. Cancer J Sci Am 1997; 3:37–44.
35. Lipford GB, Hoffman M, Wagner H, et al. Primary in vivo responses to ovalbumin. Probing the predictive value of the Kb binding motif. J Immunol 1993; 150:1212–1222.
36. Zhou FR, Rouse BT, Huang L. Prolonged survival of thymoma-bearing mice after vaccination with a soluble protein antigen entrapped in liposomes: a model study. Cancer Res 1992; 52:6287–6291.
37. Mossman SP, Evans LS, Fang H, et al. Development of a CTL vaccine for Her-2/neu using peptide-microspheres and adjuvants. Vaccine 2005; 23(27):3545–3554.
38. Zhou F, Rouse BT, Huang L. Induction of cytotoxic T lymphocytes in vivo with protein antigen entrapped in membranous vehicles. J Immunol 1992; 149:1599–1604.
39. Harty JT, Bevan MJ. CD8+ T cells specific for a single nonamer epitope of Listeria monocytogenes are protective in vivo. J Exp Med 1992; 175:1531–1538.
40. Noguchi Y, Chen YT, Old LJ. A mouse mutant p53 product recognized by CD4+ and CD8+ T cells. Proc Natl Acad Sci U S A 1994; 91:3171–3175.
41. Mayordomo JI, Zorina T, Storkus WJ, et al. Bone marrow-derived dendritic cells serve as potent adjuvants for peptide-based antitumor vaccines. Stem Cells 1997; 15:94–103.

42. Minev BR, McFarland BJ, Spiess PJ, et al. Insertion signal sequence fused to minimal peptides elicits specific CD8+ T-cell responses and prolongs survival of thymoma-bearing mice. Cancer Res 1994; 54:4155–4161.

43. Adotevi O, Mollier K, Neuveut C, et al. Immunogenic HLA-B*0702-restricted epitopes derived from human telomerase reverse transcriptase that elicit antitumor cytotoxic T-cell responses. Clin Cancer Res 2006; 12(10):3158–3167.

44. Brunsvig PF, Aamdal S, Gjertsen MK, et al. Telomerase peptide vaccination: a phase I/II study in patients with non-small cell lung cancer. Cancer Immunol Immunother 2006; 55(12):1553–1564.

45. Jager E, Ringhoffer M, Arand M, et al. Cytolytic T cell reactivity against melanoma-associated differentiation antigens in peripheral blood of melanoma patients and healthy individuals. Melanoma Res 1996; 6:419–425.

46. Rivoltini L, Kawakami Y, Sakaguchi K, et al. Induction of tumor-reactive CTL from peripheral blood and tumor-infiltrating lymphocytes of melanoma patients by in vitro stimulation with an immunodominant peptide of the human melanoma antigen MART-1. J Immunol 1995; 154(5):2257–2265.

47. Visseren MJ, van Elsas A, van der Voort EI, et al. CTL specific for the tyrosinase autoantigen can be induced from healthy donor blood to lyse melanoma cells. J Immunol 1995; 154(8):3991–3998.

48. Marchand M, Weynants P, Rankin E, et al. Tumor regression responses in melanoma patients treated with a peptide encoded by gene MAGE-3 [letter]. Int J Cancer 1995; 63:883–885.

49. Marchand M, van Baren N, Weynants P, et al. Tumor regressions observed in patients with metastatic melanoma treated with an antigenic peptide encoded by gene MAGE-3 and presented by HLA-A1. Int J Cancer 1999; 80(2):219–230.

50. Salgaller ML, Afshar A, Marincola FM, et al. Recognition of multiple epitopes in the human melanoma antigen gp100 by peripheral blood lymphocytes stimulated in vitro with synthetic peptides. Cancer Res 1995; 55:4972–4979.

51. Mukherji B, Chakraborty NG, Yamasaki S, et al. Induction of antigen-specific cytolytic T cells in situ in human melanoma by immunization with synthetic peptide-pulsed autologous antigen presenting cells. Proc Natl Acad Sci U S A 1995; 92:8078–8082.

52. Jaeger E, Bernhard H, Romero P, et al. Generation of cytotoxic T-cell responses with synthetic melanoma-associated peptides in vivo: implications for tumor vaccines with melanoma-associated antigens. Int J Cancer 1996; 66:162–169.

53. Jager E, Gnjatic S, Nagata Y, et al. Induction of primary NY-ESO-1 immunity: CD8+ T lymphocyte and antibody responses in peptide-vaccinated patients with NY-ESO-1+ cancers. PNAS 2000; 97(22):12198–12202.

54. Gjertsen MK, Bakka A, Breivik J, et al. Ex vivo ras peptide vaccination in patients with advanced pancreatic cancer: results of a phase I/II study. Int J Cancer 1996; 65:450–453.

55. Celis E. Overlapping human leukocyte antigen class I/II binding peptide vaccine for the treatment of patients with stage IV melanoma: evidence of systemic immune dysfunction. Cancer 2007; 110(1):203–214.

56. Noguchi M, Yao A, Harada M, et al. Immunological evaluation of neoadjuvant peptide vaccination before radical prostatectomy for patients with localized prostate cancer. Prostate 2007; 67(9):933–942.

57. Noguchi M, Mine T, Yamada A, et al. Combination therapy of personalized peptide vaccination and low-dose estramustine phosphate for metastatic hormone refractory

prostate cancer patients: an analysis of prognostic factors in the treatment. Oncol Res 2007; 16(7):341–349.

58. Celis E, Tsai V, Crimi C, et al. Induction of anti-tumor cytotoxic T lymphocytes in normal humans using primary cultures and synthetic peptide epitopes. Proc Natl Acad Sci U S A 1994; 91:2105–2109.

59. Vitiello A, Ishioka G, Grey HM, et al. Development of a lipopeptide-based therapeutic vaccine to treat chronic HBV infection. I. Induction of a primary cytotoxic T lymphocyte response in humans. J Clin Invest 1995; 95:341–349.

60. Sette A, Alexander J, Ruppert J, et al. Antigen analogs/MHC complexes as specific T cell receptor antagonists. Annu Rev Immunol 1994; 12:413–431.

61. Parkhurst MR, Salgaller ML, Southwood S, et al. Improved induction of melanoma-reactive CTL with peptides from the melanoma antigen gp100 modified at HLA-A*0201-binding residues. J Immunol 1996; 157:2539–2548.

62. Eguchi J, Hatano M, Nishimura F, et al. Identification of interleukin-13 receptor alpha2 peptide analogues capable of inducing improved antiglioma CTL responses. Cancer Res 2006; 66(11):5883–5891.

63. Phan GQ, Yang JC, Sherry RM, et al. Cancer regression and autoimmunity induced by cytotoxic T lymphocyte-associated antigen 4 blockade in patients with metastatic melanoma. Proc Natl Acad Sci U S A 2003; 100(14):8372–8377.

64. Sanderson K, Scotland R, Lee P, et al. Autoimmunity in a phase I trial of a fully human anti-cytotoxic T-lymphocyte antigen-4 monoclonal antibody with multiple melanoma peptides and Montanide ISA 51 for patients with resected stages III and IV melanoma. J Clin Oncol 2005; 23(4):741–750.

65. Wang F, Bade E, Kuniyoshi C, et al. Phase I trial of a MART-1 peptide vaccine with incomplete Freund's adjuvant for resected high-risk melanoma. Clin Cancer Res 1999; 5(10):2756–2765.

66. Jeager E, Maeurer M, Heohn H, et al. Clonal expansion of Melan A-specific cytotoxic T lymphocytes in a melanoma patient responding to continued immunization with melanoma-associated peptides. Int J Cancer 2000; 86(4):538–547.

67. Brinckerhoff LH, Kalashnikov VV, Thompson LW, et al. Terminal modifications inhibit proteolytic degradation of an immunogenic MART-1(27-35) peptide: implications for peptide vaccines. Int J Cancer 1999; 83(3):326–334.

68. Minev BR, Chavez FL, Dudouet BM, et al. Synthetic insertion signal sequences enhance MHC class I presentation of a peptide from the melanoma antigen MART-1. Eur J Immunol 2000; 30:2115–2124.

69. Anderson K, Cresswell P, Gammon M, et al. Endogenously synthesized peptide with an endoplasmic reticulum signal sequence sensitizes antigen processing mutant cells to class I-restricted cell-mediated lysis. J Exp Med 1991; 174:489–492.

70. Okada CY, Rechsteiner M. Introduction of macromolecules into cultured mammalian cells by osmotic lysis of pinocytic vesicles. Cell 1982; 29:33–41.

71. Persson H, Jornvall H, Zabielski J. Multiple mRNA species for the precursor to an adenovirus-encoded glycoprotein: identification and structure of the signal sequence. Proc Natl Acad Sci U S A 1980; 77:6349–6353.

72. Houghton M, Stewart AG, Doel SM, et al. The amino-terminal sequence of human fibroblast interferon as deduced from reverse transcripts obtained using synthetic oligonucleotide primers. Nucleic Acids Res 1980; 8:1913–1931.

73. Heemels MT, Ploegh H. Generation, translocation, and presentation of MHC class I-restricted peptides. Annu Rev Biochem 1995; 64:463–491.

74. Restifo NP, Esquivel F, Kawakami Y, et al. Identification of human cancers deficient in antigen processing. J Exp Med 1993; 177:265–272.

75. Slingluff CL Jr., Petroni GR, Yamshchikov GV, et al. Immunologic and clinical outcomes of vaccination with a multiepitope melanoma peptide vaccine plus low-dose interleukin-2 administered either concurrently or on a delayed schedule. J Clin Oncol 2004; 22(22):4474–4485.

76. Lee P, Wang F, Kuniyoshi J, et al. Effects of interleukin-12 on the immune response to a multipeptide vaccine for resected metastatic melanoma. J Clin Oncol 2001; 19(18):3836–3847.

77. Peterson AC, Harlin H, Gajewski TF. Immunization with Melan-A peptide-pulsed peripheral blood mononuclear cells plus recombinant human interleukin-12 induces clinical activity and T-cell responses in advanced melanoma. J Clin Oncol 2003; 21(12):2342–2348.

78. Chianese-Bullock KA, Pressley J, Garbee C, et al. MAGE-A1-, MAGE-A10-, and gp100-derived peptides are immunogenic when combined with granulocyte-macro-phage colony-stimulating factor and montanide ISA-51 adjuvant and administered as part of a multipeptide vaccine for melanoma. J Immunol 2005; 174(5):3080–3086.

79. Hersey P, Menzies SW, Coventry B, et al. Phase I/II study of immunotherapy with T-cell peptide epitopes in patients with stage IV melanoma. Cancer Immunol Immunother 2005; 54(3):208–218.

80. Pullarkat V, Lee PP, Scotland R, et al. A phase I trial of SD-9427 (progenipoietin) with a multipeptide vaccine for resected metastatic melanoma. Clin Cancer Res 2003; 9(4):1301–1312.

81. Butterfield LH, Ribas A, Meng WS, et al. T-cell responses to HLA-A*0201 immunodominant peptides derived from alpha-fetoprotein in patients with hep-atocellular cancer. Clin Cancer Res 2003; 9(16 pt 1):5902–5908.

82. Vonderheide RH, Domchek SM, Schultze JL, et al. Vaccination of cancer patients against telomerase induces functional antitumor CD8+ T lymphocytes. Clin Cancer Res 2004; 10(3):828–839.

83. McNeel DG, Knutson KL, Schiffman K, et al. Pilot study of an HLA-A2 peptide vaccine using flt3 ligand as a systemic vaccine adjuvant. J Clin Immunol 2003; 23(1):62–72.

84. Hueman MT, Stojadinovic A, Storrer CE, et al. Levels of circulating regulatory CD4+CD25+ T cells are decreased in breast cancer patients after vaccination with a HER2/neu peptide (E75) and GM-CSF vaccine. Breast Cancer Res Treat 2006; 98(1): 17–29.

85. Hueman MT, Stojadinovic A, Storrer CE, et al. Analysis of naive and memory CD4 and CD8 T cell populations in breast cancer patients receiving a HER2/neu peptide (E75) and GM-CSF vaccine. Cancer Immunol Immunother 2007; 56(2):135–146.

86. Davila E, Kennedy R, Celis E. Generation of antitumor immunity by cytotoxic T lymphocyte epitope peptide vaccination, CpG-oligodeoxynucleotide adjuvant, and CTLA-4 blockade. Cancer Res 2003; 63(12):3281–3288.

87. Celis E, Sette A, Grey HM. Epitope selection and development of peptide based vaccines to treat cancer. Semin Cancer Biol 1995; 6:329–336.

88. Itoh K, Yamada A. Personalized peptide vaccines: a new therapeutic modality for cancer. Cancer Sci 2006; 97(10):970–976.

89. Nowak MA, May RM, Phillips RE, et al. Antigenic oscillations and shifting immunodominance in HIV-1 infections [see comments]. Nature 1995; 375:606–611.

90. Toes RE, Offringa R, Blom RJ, et al. Peptide vaccination can lead to enhanced tumor growth through specific T-cell tolerance induction. Proc Natl Acad Sci U S A 1996; 93:7855–7860.

91. Webb S, Morris C, Sprent J. Extrathymic tolerance of mature T cells: clonal elimination as a consequence of immunity. Cell 1990; 63:1249–1256.

92. Aichele P, Brduscha-Riem K, Zinkernagel RM, et al. T cell priming versus T cell tolerance induced by synthetic peptides. J Exp Med 1995; 182:261–266.

93. Benichou G, Fedoseyeva E, Olson CA, et al. Disruption of the determinant hierarchy on a self-MHC peptide: concomitant tolerance induction to the dominant determinant and priming to the cryptic self-determinant. Int Immunol 1994; 6:131–138.

94. Sercarz EE, Lehmann PV, Ametani A, et al. Dominance and crypticity of T cell antigenic determinants. Annu Rev Immunol 1993; 11:729–766.

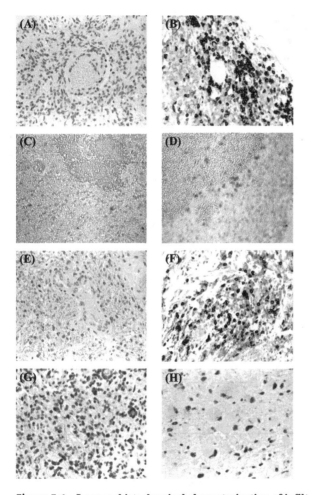

Figure 5.1   Immunohistochemical characterization of infiltrating cells in intracranial tumor before and after DC vaccination: Intratumoral CD8$^+$ cells, pre- (**A**), and post-vaccination (**B**). Intratumoral CD4$^+$ cells, pre- (**C**), and post-vaccination (**D**). Intratumoral CD45RO$^+$ cells, pre- (**E**), and post-vaccination (**F**). Intratumoral CD8$^+$ cells pre- (**G**) and post-recurrence (**H**) in a non-vaccinated patient.

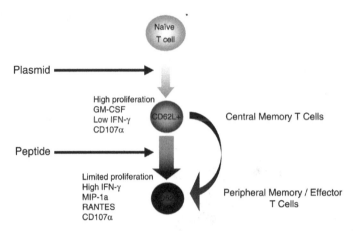

Figure 7.3 Hypothetic events during DNA priming, peptide-boosting immunization regimen in the LN. Plasmid-driven antigen expression within secondary lymphoid organs promotes a central (CD62L$^+$) memory T-cell population capable of rapid and substantial expansion. Exposure to peptide triggers a preferential proliferation of CD62L$^+$ cells as well as the loss of CD62L expression resulting in the significant shift from a more balanced CD62L$^+$ and CD62L$^-$ to a more pronounced CD62L$^-$ phenotype of specific T-cell population after peptide boost. In parallel, a redistribution of CD8$^+$ T cells between lymphoid and nonlymphoid organs is evident, together with the acquisition of IFN-γ and chemokine expression capability by CD62L CD8$^+$ T cells. Both central and peripheral CD8$^+$ T cells show de-granulation (CD107alpha upregulation) upon peptide stimulation. *Abbreviations*: LN, lymph node; IFN, interferon.

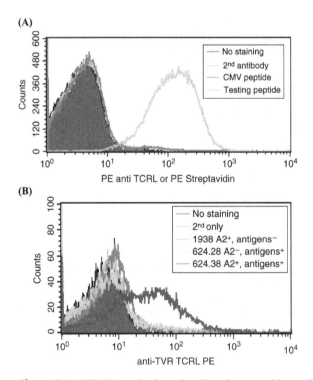

Figure 9.1 TCR-like antibody against Tyrosinase peptide specifically recognizes Tyrosinase 369–377/HLA-A2 complex on **(A)** peptide-loaded JY cells and **(B)** Tyrosinase expressing, HLA-A2 tumor cell line Mel 624.38.

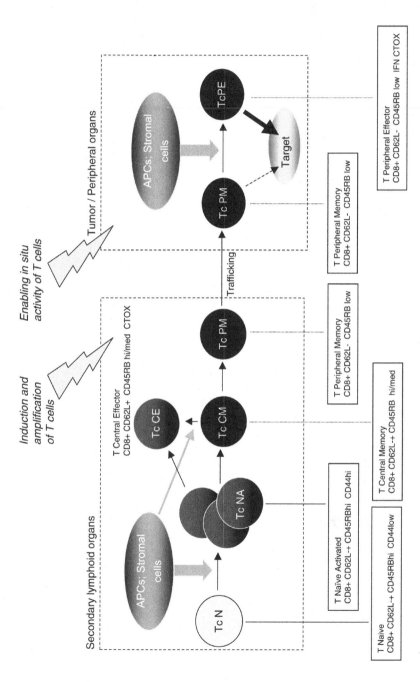

Figure 8.5 A schematic representation of induction, expansion, differentiation, and migration of tumor antigen–specific T cells upon vaccination against tumor-associated antigens. *Abbreviations:* TcN, T cytotoxic naive; Tc NA, Tc naive activated; Tc CM, Tc central memory; Tc CE, Tc effectors; Tc PM, Tc peripheral memory; Tc PE, Tc peripheral effectors.

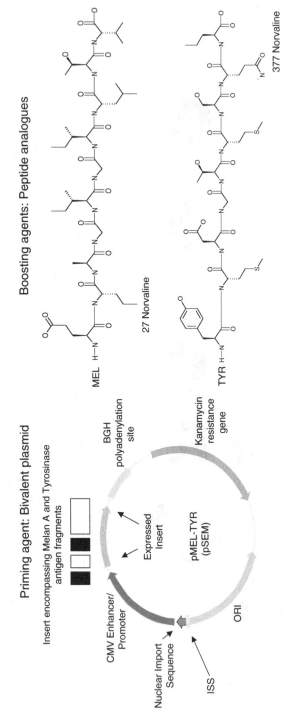

Figure 8.14 Schematic representation of a multicomponent investigational agent encompassing a plasmid vector and two peptide analogues.

Multimodality Immunization Approaches to Improve on DNA Vaccines for Cancer

Zhiyong Qiu and Kent A. Smith

*Division of Translational Medicine, MannKind Corporation,
Valencia, California, U.S.A.*

INTRODUCTION

The discovery, more than a decade ago, that naked plasmid vectors expressing exogenous genes can be utilized to elicit immune responses promoted an unprecedented excitement and pursue of this strategy in preclinical and clinical development of innovative biotherapeutics in infectious diseases (1–3), cancer (4–7), and autoimmunity (8–10). An initial momentum resulting from promising preclinical results has been somewhat diminished subsequently due to modest efficacy data obtained in various clinical trials, particularly in prophylactic settings (11,12). Nevertheless, features such as the apparent simplicity of mechanism of action, intrinsic adjuvant properties, favorable safety profile, and ease in manufacturing, all warrant a careful analysis of the limiting factors associated with DNA vaccination with the purpose of designing novel strategies that leverage these beneficial features.

One of the hallmarks of plasmid immunization is that the antigen-presenting cells (APCs) have relatively prolonged exposure to low levels of antigen. While this may lead to the generation of high-quality responses, it has been difficult to obtain high-magnitude responses using such vaccines, even with repeated booster doses, a phenomenon likely due to the relatively low levels of epitope loading onto major histocompatibility complex (MHC) achieved with these vectors. Various prime-boost strategies have been developed, aiming at amplifying the high-quality response generated during the DNA priming interval, including the use of proteins (13,14) or live virus vectors (15,16). Such approaches are generally successful in inducing protective immunity against microbial or tumorigenic viruses; however, it is much more difficult to generate responses at the magnitude of therapeutic usefulness to tumor antigens.

Unlike prophylactic vaccination aimed at priming the immune system with an antigen that has never been encountered, tumor antigens are self-antigens that are expressed during early development or disease stage, resulting in immune tolerance to these antigens. Removal or silencing of high-avidity, self-reactive T cells to ubiquitously expressed or blood-borne antigens from the repertoire in thymus is necessary to prevent autoimmunity, a mechanism known as central tolerance (reviewed in Ref. 17). In addition, peripheral tolerance involving a multitude of factors contributes to the suppression of T-cell functions toward tissue-restricted antigens. Therefore, therapeutic cancer vaccines need to overcome the hurdle of immune tolerance to induce immune responses of high quantity as well as high quality in order to achieve positive clinical outcomes. While more stringent requirements for activation and effector function are necessary for lower avidity T-cell precursors, a successful cancer vaccine should also be capable of directing T cells to traffic out of the lymphoid organs and migrating to the tumor sites where tumor-specific recognition and immune attack take place. Various experimental models have been established in the last decade, and in this chapter, we outline the pros and cons of those models emphasizing the prime-boost immunization approaches using plasmid vectors based on understanding of the mechanism of action and options to build superior immunization strategies.

DNA IMMUNIZATION: MECHANISMS OF ACTION

Many studies were carried out in preclinical models, to address the mechanism of action of DNA immunization, employing quite diverse and creative designs. Most notably, use of bone marrow chimeric (BMC) mice, adoptive cell transfer, strategies of identification and tracking of in situ transfected somatic cells or APCs, manipulation of immune costimulation, and evaluation of the role of innate immune cells, all contributed to the emergence of multiple models explaining the induction of immunity subsequent to DNA vector administration (Fig. 1).

The majority of earlier studies were carried out by intramuscular injection of plasmid, which conclusively showed the in situ expression of transgene within myocytes (18). It is estimated that hundreds, or at the maximum thousands, of myocytes acquired transgene expression that usually lasted for days/ weeks—parameters sufficing the induction of a class I–restricted immune response (19–22). Transplantation of ex vivo transfected myocytes and measurement of immunity in BMC mice demonstrated the necessity of matched MHC

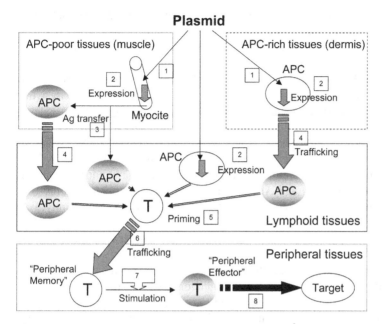

Figure 1 Factors impacting the efficacy of plasmids as vaccines or immunotherapeutics
(1). In vivo transfection of somatic and bone marrow–derived APCs occurs in a fashion
depending on route of administration. While intramuscular injection results in prepon-
derent transfection of myocytes, intradermal injection results in transfection of significant
numbers of Langerhans cells with LN-migrating capabilities (2). In situ transfected
somatic or APCs express differentially the plasmid-borne transgene, both quantitatively as
well as from a temporal aspect. Overall however, the number of cells expressing the
plasmid transgene in situ ranges from tens to thousands, with expression lasting a few
days only, if administration is not repeated (3). Antigen or plasmid transfer from
somatically transfected cells to APCs is a key limiting event in case of intramuscular
administration of plasmid and may occur in the form of HSP-peptide complexes or other
yet undefined mechanisms (4). APC trafficking to the draining LNs is another key
event, facilitated by the migrating capabilities of in situ transfected APCs and followed
by (5) priming of naïve T cells within germinal centers of secondary lymphoid organs
(6). The process of primary expansion of T cells and subsequent differentiation is
guided by the molecular microenvironment within the lymphoid node, shaping up the
nature of the resulting central and peripheral memory cells (7). The peripheral memory
cells have the capability to surveil nonlymphoid organs and display residual effector
functions, and (8) can acquire additional ones upon interaction with immune-stimulating
factors within the target organ (9). Finally, target cells (tumoral or viral infected) are acted
upon by effector T cells in a fashion depending on a variety of factors. *Abbreviations*: LN,
lymph nodes; HSP, heat shock protein; APC, antigen-presenting cell.

restriction, between bone marrow–derived APCs and T cells (20–23). However, such identical MHC allele is not required between antigen-expressing myocytes and T cells together (23); the ample evidence accumulated in this regard challenged the somewhat simplistic view that in situ transfected cells are directly priming specific T cells. Instead, there must be antigen transfer between in situ transfected myocytes and APCs, with subsequent priming of T cells within secondary lymphoid organs (cross-priming). Only more recently, accumulated evidence suggests that the antigen transfer between in situ transfected somatic cells and APCs may occur in the form of heat shock protein (HSP)-polypeptide complexes and is facilitated by the apoptosis of transgene-expressing cells (24,25). However, it is highly likely that there is a multiplicity of mechanisms accounting for the antigen transfer between myocytes and APCs, and they may have different bearings on induction of cytotoxic T lymphocytes (CTL) versus other types of immunity. For example, engineering export sequences within the open reading frame of the plasmid vector resulted in increased Th and B cell responses, without a similar effect on the CTL response suggesting that antigen transfer as secreted protein, between myocytes and APCs, results in effective handling via the exogenous, but not the MHC class I processing and presentation, pathway (26). Overall, such elegant studies—coupled with the scarcity or lack of transgene-expressing APCs—contributed to a momentum behind the cross-priming/cross-processing model.

Nevertheless, interestingly, a series of reports obtained in slightly different experimental setups challenged the cross-priming model. For example, it was demonstrated that intradermal plasmid injection results in coexpression of the transgene by somatic cells and APCs and that upon adoptive transfer of migrating APCs, an increased MHC class I–restricted immune response is elicited (27). Mere antigen transfer between somatic cells and APCs was ruled out by using plasmids expressing antigens encompassing nuclear import sequences (28), in conjunction with multicolor, high-resolution cell-imaging techniques. Innovative approaches to administer plasmid vectors to the dermis by gene gun or other strategies showed that much lower doses were needed to elicit an immune response, compared to more traditional intramuscular administration (29). An emerging model shaped up, by which in situ transfected Langerhans cells, upon migration to the draining lymph node (LN), actually prime specific T cells utilizing the conventional processing pathway (reviewed in Ref. 30).

The apparent conundrum relative to the importance of cross-priming versus conventional pathway of induction of MHC class I–restricted immunity by plasmid immunization can be addressed by judging the experimental evidence in light of the route and strategy of administration. The key parameter in this regard is the presence and the density of competent APCs within the injected tissue, capable of expressing the transgene, migrating to draining LN and priming specific T cells (30,31). While both the conventional and cross-priming mechanisms take place simultaneously, their relative importance is fundamentally different as follows: In case of intramuscular injection, the scarcity of resident APCs determines a near-exclusive reliance on cross-priming—except when strategies to increase the influx of APCs are deployed (32). In contrast, injection of plasmid into dendritic cell (DC)-rich areas such as dermis results in the induction of MHC class I– restricted immunity via conventional processing and priming pathways (29,30). The relative potential of these pathways is suggested by dose-effect, adoptive cell-transfer experiments, in which in situ transfected professional APCs and somatic cells, respectively, were separately infused in naïve mice. While non-APCs yielded a limited immune response, the transgene-expressing, professional APCs induced a significantly increased response (29) illustrating the concept that in the course of DNA immunization, the conventional processing/priming pathway has a higher potential from this standpoint, as compared to cross-processing/cross-priming. This has been strongly supported by reports showing that direct intra-splenic or LN administration of naked plasmid resulted in increased immunity, as assessed in a dose-effect fashion (33). It is likely that targeted administration of naked plasmid to APC-rich tissues results in increased numbers of competent APCs presenting the antigen directly to specific T cells, even if the overall number of host cells effectively transfected is not superior over those achieved by intra-muscular or subcutaneous administration. In fact, a recent study provided further support to this concept by demonstrating that the use of a device to increase the exposure of dermal APCs to plasmid vaccine, as opposed to conventional bolus injection, resulted in increased immunity (34). Strikingly, despite the fact that intramuscular injection resulted in higher antigen expression for a prolonged interval (weeks), intradermal administration using a tattoo device resulted in a relatively reduced antigen expression over only a few days; however, it was far more effective in inducing T-cell immunity (35).

The multiplicity of mechanisms by which plasmids elicit immune responses, depending on the route of administration and other factors, results in a number of limiting steps relative to the magnitude of the resulting immune response (Fig. 1). These can be thus addressed by various means, as listed in Table 1. More important, addressing limiting factors on individual basis may not be enough to effectively improve the potency of DNA vaccines; instead, significantly superior strategies must troubleshoot as many as possible, if not all, rate-limiting factors.

ADVANTAGES OF PLASMID VECTORS AS THERAPEUTIC VACCINES FOR CANCER

Among different vaccine forms for treating cancer, DNA vaccine has several advantages such as immunogenicity, intrinsic adjuvant effect, capacity for harboring larger or multiple antigens and ease to manipulate, preferred safety profile, excellent stability, and inexpensive manufacturing cost.

The cellular arm of the immune response, the focus of active immunotherapy employing DNA vaccination, results from uptake of plasmids into cells (DCs, Langerhans cells, and muscle cells) (30,31), where the encoding target

Table 1 Multimodality Heterologous Prime-Boost Immunization in Clinic

Disease category	Targeted antigen	Priming agent	Boosting agent	Immune responses	Clinical responses	References
Infectious diseases	HIV gag	DNA	MVA	T cell response (8/9)	Not available	46
	HIV gp120	Canarypox virus	Gp120 protein	Neutralizing Ab-induced poor T-cell response	Not available	47
	HIV gag pol and env	DNA	Adenovirus	Not available	Not available	
	Malaria TRAP	DNA	MVA	CD4 and CD8 persistence of immune response for months	Partial protection	48
Cancer	NY-ESO-1	Recombinant vaccinia or poxvirus	Recombinant vaccinia or poxvirus	Ab, CD4, and CD8	Favorable clinical outcome	49
	Multiple epitopes for melanoma	DNA	MVA	Biased T-cell response (against 1/7 epitope)	Not available	50
	PSA	Recombinant vaccinia or poxvirus	Recombinant vaccinia or poxvirus	46% of subjects have increase in PSA-reactive T cells	Not significant	51
	CEA	Recombinant vaccinia	Recombinant poxvirus	6/6 subjects have increase in frequency of T cells	No objective antitumor response	52

Abbreviation: MVA, vaccinia virus Ankara.

antigen is expressed. The resulting proteins undergo proteolytic processing in the proteasomes, producing peptides that bind to class I MHC molecules. The presentation of these MHC-bound peptides on the cell surface of APCs stimulates $CD8^+$ CTL response. Results from preclinical studies and clinical trials have also indicated that the route of administration and the dosage used are critical in the induction of immune responses, involving different mechanism of actions (Fig. 1). Immune responses from intramuscular administration of plasmid DNA are largely dependent on cross-priming, the mechanism of which is yet to be understood. Novel approaches have been explored in directly targeting APCs, especially DCs (36–38). As will be discussed below, naked plasmid DNA combined with the prime-boost immunization regimen may be a very attractive way to prime high-affinity and high-avidity CTL responses.

For therapeutic vaccine against cancer, targeting multiple CD8-specific epitopes derived from different tumor antigens (as opposed to monovalent approaches) is believed to be more effective, considering the heterogeneity and genetic instability of tumor cells (39). Plasmid can naturally harbor larger DNA fragments of coding sequences, thus making it possible to express in vivo engineered synthetic tumor antigen. Prophylactic and therapeutic vaccines expressing polyepitope strings have been tested in clinical settings, and responses were observed for multiple epitopes in the string (40–42), indicating that these epitopes are successfully processed and presented in humans. However, in order to achieve optimal and balanced immune responses for each epitope with intrinsic immunological properties, it is necessary to modify coding sequences in the plasmid. This can be achieved by simple manipulations in the expression insert followed by direct assessment of immunogenicity of vaccines after direct injection of the plasmid DNA. Such methodology will greatly enhance our ability for rational vaccine design as well as further our understanding of molecular basis of the immune response.

PRIME-BOOST STRATEGIES IN CANCER IMMUNOTHERAPY

Immunization has traditionally relied on repeated administration of antigen to augment the magnitude of the immune response. With the advancement in recombinant DNA technology, genetically engineered vaccines such as expression plasmids, recombinant proteins, viruses, and bacteria have become the latest modalities for vaccine development. The first such vaccine in its class, a hepatitis B virus vaccine in the form of recombinant protein produced in yeast, has been shown to be potent in providing protective efficacy in humans (43,44). While this homologous protein-based immunization is very effective for generating humoral immune responses, it is generally inefficient in inducing cell-mediated immunity important for protection against infections caused by intracellular pathogens and for cancer immunotherapy. DNA vaccines, on the other hand, have been tested in small and large animal models, and have demonstrated efficacy in inducing both humoral and cellular immunity for infectious diseases and cancer, while clinical trials of such DNA vaccines have provided mixed results (45). In parallel with the development of DNA vaccines, recombinant viral vectors, such as poxviruses and adenoviruses, have emerged as vaccine delivery systems. In mice as well as nonhuman primates, recombinant viral vectors are very efficient for the induction of cellular and humoral immunity, characterized by increased $CD4^+$ and $CD8^+$ T cells as well as antibodies. However, DNA vaccines or recombinant viral vectors failed to induce the high levels of antigen-specific T cells necessary for protection against intracellular pathogens when used singly or with repeated administration (homologous boosting). This has led to the investigation of whether heterologous prime-boost immunizations with different modalities can elicit immune responses of greater magnitude and quality than can be achieved by priming and boosting with the same vector.

It has been well established that cellular immunity is the key in controlling tumorigenesis and microbial infections of intracellular pathogen that involves induction and expansion of antigen-specific T cells endowed with multiple capabilities such as migration, effector functions, and differentiation into memory cells. Earlier studies attempted to elucidate the sequence and combination of modalities during a heterologous prime-boost immunization regimen that results in the generation of antigen-specific memory T cells by priming followed by amplification of these cells by boosting. A variety of such vaccine components have been evaluated in preclinical models or human trials including DNA plasmid, recombinant poxviruses and adenoviruses, alphavirus replicon particles, modified vaccinia virus Ankara, and protein or peptide in adjuvants. Results from these studies revealed that multiple mechanisms account for the efficiency of prime-boost vaccination protocols; however, synergy in epitope presentation during priming and boosting by different expression vectors is the key requirement to evoke high-avidity CD8 cells in the host, while additive effect may result from other features within the boosting vector. Table 1 summarizes some major findings from such studies in humans.

DNA vaccines have been widely accepted as good priming agents since they can trigger antigen presentation via both MHC class I and class II, thereby inducing both CTL and Th1 lymphocytes via a mechanism of action depicted in Figure 1. To leverage the high quality of the immune response primed by plasmid DNA and likely facilitated by its excellent toll-like receptors 9 (TLR9)-dependent and -independent adjuvant activities, various groups have explored boosting strategies by delivery of targeted antigen incorporated in different forms. Such boosting components encompass proteins, live viral vectors, or plasmid vectors. There is an extensive database obtained in preclinical models and in clinics supporting this concept, mostly in the area of prophylactic immunization for infectious diseases targeting pathogens such as HIV (13), malaria (53), and tuberculosis (54). Priming with plasmid DNA and boosting with live vector has shown, by far, to be the most effective regimen to induce immune response at the level of therapeutic usefulness both in preclinical and in clinical trials (46,48,55,56). For cancer immunotherapy, a pioneer work a decade ago by Irvine et al. showed that heterologous prime-boost strategy can augment antitumor immunity by generating a strong antigen-specific CTL response in mice (57). Their data suggested that immunizing with DNA and boosting with a live viral vector expressing the same tumor-associated antigen prolonged the survival of tumor-bearing mice more efficiently than multiple immunizations with the same vector, correlating with stronger specific CTL responses (57). Meng et al. performed a similar study on mice by administration of plasmid DNA encoding murine α-fetoprotein followed by boosting with a nonreplicating adenoviral vector expressing the same antigen (58). This immunization strategy resulted in elicitation of high frequency of Th1-type α-fetoprotein-specific cells leading to tumor protective immunity in mice at levels comparable with α-fetoprotein-engineered DCs (58). However, in clinic, data from a phase I trial of sequential administration of plasmid DNA and adenovirus expressing L523S protein in patients with early-stage non-small-cell lung cancer showed a high level of safety but limited evidence of L523S-directed immune activation (59), suggesting that a further optimized immunization approach is needed to break immune tolerance or ignorance to self-antigens.

Despite the mounting data demonstrating the tolerability of live vectors in preventive vaccination, there is significant safety concern for the use of such vectors in cancer patients who may be at the stage of immune suppression after prolonged chemotherapy. Additional drawbacks of the use of live viral vectors include antibody responses to vectors that diminish effectiveness of later boosts, and higher development and production costs. Therefore, considerable efforts have been devoted to explore nonviral options for boosting immunity generated during the DNA-priming interval. DNA vector itself has been shown to induce suboptimal immunity even after repeated immunization. However, the use of DNA vectors with a modified sequence, or delivered in a different mechanism, as a boosting agent, lead to a significantly improved immune response. Preclinical animal models have demonstrated that the use of an "altered self" form of antigen may provide $CD4^+$ T cell help to break the tolerance and to induce tumor protection (60). Such hypothesis is further tested in mice with a prime-boost immunization regimen with plasmids expressing human or mouse tyrosinase-related protein 1 (TRP-1) (60). That priming with human TRP-1 DNA broke tolerance to mouse TRP-1 was evidenced by the manifestations of autoimmunity, characterized by coat depigmentation, and such immune responses to TRP-1 provided significant protection against colonization of the lung by metastatic melanoma cells (60). The presence of slight differences in epitopes between host "self" protein and that encoded by xenogeneic DNA plasmid vaccine, along with inherent bacterial unmethylated CpG motifs, may be sufficient to boost the immune response to break tolerance and ignorance to tumors. Currently, such approaches are in clinical proof of principle testing with two well-defined tumor antigens-prostate-specific membrane antigen and tyrosinase (61,62). Another approach is priming with naked DNA and boosting with the same vector in combination with the use of an electroporation device to improve the immune responses. In both animal and clinical trials with prophylactic DNA vaccines, electroporation enhances immune responses to DNA vaccines by increasing gene expression as well as inducing inflammatory cell infiltration (63). Such strategy has also been explored in cancer with two tumor models, the CT26 carcinoma

Table 2 Advantages of Plasmid Vectors as Vaccines

Features	Mechanism of action/rationale
Induction of broad immune responses encompassing MHC class I–restricted T cells	Direct transfection of APCs and/or cross-presentation
Predominant induction of T1 immune responses	Binding to TLRs and activation of dependent innate immune pathways
Beneficial safety profile	Lack of replication, transient, episomal persistence, infrequent genomic integration
Simplicity of manufacturing	Straightforward *E. Coli* fermentation process and plasmid purification

Abbreviations: APCs, antigen-presenting cells; MHC, major histocompatibility complex; TLR, toll-like receptors.

and the BCL1 lymphoma (64,65). It is interesting to note that for such homologous prime-boost approach, the most effective way to generate a potent immune response is priming with naked plasmid DNA and boosting with the same vector using an electroporation device. The mechanism of improved immune response by electroporation of vaccine plasmids during boosting is still not completely understood; however, it involves at least two features, namely, increased antigen expression and necrosis at the injection site, which induce inflammation. It is also possible that in electroporated APCs, an elevated antigen expression may also introduce a subtle shift of antigen presentation, a slight different processing compared to that of cells in vivo transfected with naked DNA, providing additional CD4$^+$ T cell help (Table 2).

Other nonviral vectors such as the simplest ones, namely, the peptides, generally have a poor pharmacokinetics profile. Recently, it was shown that intra-LN injection of T-cell epitope peptides may actually circumvent their poor pharmacokinetics and leverage their intrinsic immune properties (66). More significantly, plasmid priming and peptide boosting achieved extremely robust immune responses (nearly 1/5 CD8$^+$ T cells specific for a given epitope; Fig. 2) in a preclinical model consisting of immunization of HLA-A2 transgenic mice (67) immunized against Melan A antigen. Not unexpectedly, this outcome could be achieved only by intra-LN administration of both plasmid and peptide rather than subcutaneous injection, reinforcing the importance of targeted delivery for the purpose of accessing APCs. In addition, with such a high number of epitope-specific CD8 cells, it becomes feasible to delineate the functional role of vectors by defining the phenotype of specific T-cell population during priming and boosting. By using cell separation techniques, multicolor FACS analysis, and ex vivo functional evaluation, it has been demonstrated that while plasmid priming generated both central and peripheral memory T cells, peptide boosting had a

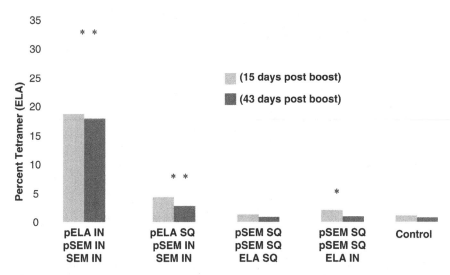

Figure 2 Comparison between the immune responses achieved by intra-LN and subcutaneous injection of plasmid and peptide in a plasmid prime–peptide boost fashion. Equivalent dosage, 25 μg of plasmid (pSEM) or peptide (Melan A 26–35 analogue) in 25 μL of sterile PBS, was administered to HHD transgenic mice via the intranodal injected and/or administrated in subcutaneous route. The number of injections remained the same. The results were expressed as percent tetramer$^+$ CD8$^+$ T cells within the CD8$^+$ T cell population, measured in blood, at 15 days after the completion of the immunization protocol (mean ± SEM; n = five mice per group). *Abbreviations*: LN, lymph nodes; PBS, phosphate-buffered saline.

profound impact in differentiation and relative expansion of CD62L$^-$ peripheral memory CD8$^+$ T cells. The latter was paralleled by migration of CD8$^+$ T cells out of LNs to nonlymphoid organs, along with a gain of function for interferon (IFN)-γ and chemokine expression, a key feature of peripheral memory/effector T cells. Figure 3 depicts a model of the prime-boost approach and the impact of plasmid and peptide on various T-cell subsets, respectively.

STRATEGIES TO IMRPOVE EFFICACY OF DNA VACCINE

Clinical trials with DNA vaccines expressing microbial antigens showed a favorable safety profile, but a relatively modest immune response, and thus moderated the initial enthusiasm in regard to this new approach for immunization (45). Various factors may have contributed in concert, to the apparent discrepancy between the generally exciting preclinical results and the modest clinical data: (1) predominant use of the intramuscular administration route, relying on cross-processing as a main mechanism of action (MOA); (2) relatively diminished inoculation volumes and amounts relative to the body mass;

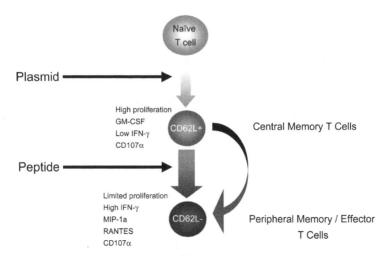

Figure 3 (*See color insert.*) Hypothetic events during DNA priming, peptide-boosting immunization regimen in the LN. Plasmid-driven antigen expression within secondary lymphoid organs promotes a central (CD62L$^+$) memory T-cell population capable of rapid and substantial expansion. Exposure to peptide triggers a preferential proliferation of CD62L$^+$ cells as well as the loss of CD62L expression resulting in the significant shift from a more balanced CD62L$^+$ and CD62L$^-$ to a more pronounced CD62L$^-$ phenotype of specific T-cell population after peptide boost. In parallel, a redistribution of CD8$^+$ T cells between lymphoid and nonlymphoid organs is evident, together with the acquisition of IFN-γ and chemokine expression capability by CD62L CD8$^+$ T cells. Both central and peripheral CD8$^+$ T cells show de-granulation (CD107alpha upregulation) upon peptide stimulation. *Abbreviations*: LN, lymph node; IFN, interferon.

(3) possible species-specific recognition of unmethylated CpG motifs; and (4) use of different methods to measure the immune response, leading to overestimation of preclinical results (for example, utilization of ultra-sensitive assays, encompassing ex vivo expansion of T cells, in case of preclinical studies; in contrast, reliance on less refined but probably more realistic readouts in case of clinical studies).

Based on these observations, many strategies have been and are currently being tested at various stages of research and development, aimed at trouble-shooting the limitations of naked plasmids as vaccines: The simplest ones were the complementation of DNA vaccines via prime-boost approaches or the use of synthetic CpG motifs as adjuvants, the utilization of electroporation or trans-fection-enhancing techniques, the use of targeted approaches such as intradermal via gene gun devices, development of new vectors expressing larger amounts of antigen, or coadministration of vectors expressing antigen and cytokines.

Consistent with the fact that the number of antigen-expressing cells was a limiting factor relative to the magnitude of immune response as shown by adoptive transfer experiments employing various numbers of in situ transfected

Langerhans cells (29), direct plasmid administration into LNs resulted in significantly superior CTL responses in a preclinical model (38). Thus, lower doses of plasmid were sufficient to induce a measurable response, as compared to intramuscular immunization—a situation somewhat reminiscent of gene gun vaccination. However, interestingly, there was little evidence that the overall magnitude of response (at plateau or saturation) was different (Table 3).

Table 3 Limiting Factors Associated with DNA Immunization and Strategies to Address Those

Limiting factors	Strategies to improve on efficacy
Limited number of in situ transfected host cells	Electroporation, use of transfection-enhancing reagents, intralymphatic injection of plasmid
Limited timeframe of plasmid expression	Repeated administration, infusion, interference with gene-silencing mechanisms
Antigen transfer to APCs, particularly if injection occurs into tissues lacking APCs	Increase apoptosis of in situ transfected somatic cells, use of export sequences, engineered HSP-antigen constructs
APC migration to LNs	Use of plasmids loaded with immune-stimulating sequences; circumvent this process by direct intra-LN injection
T-cell priming, limited by the reduced number of APCs within germinal centers	Provision of balanced antigen and costimulating signals, over a key time interval
Expansion and differentiation of T cells, influenced by activation of innate immunity and antigen exposure within LN	Complement plasmid priming with boost strategies using alternate vectors; provide effective innate immune stimulation
T-cell trafficking and immune surveillance, enabled by T-cell differentiation and loss of LN homing receptors	Provide effective costimulation, use of appropriate dosages, immunization protocols, thereby avoiding induction of anergy or tolerance; targeted delivery of chemoattractants
Acquisition and maintenance of effector functions by T cells, influenced by the LN and target organ microenvironment	Interfere with induction of T regulatory cells, control of target organ microenvironment by administration of proinflammatory agents
Target cell destruction, dependent on the avidity of TCR for the MHC-peptide complex, along with other factors	Use of epitope analogues to elicit improved T-cell immunity against self-epitopes; improve on the antigenicity of target cells (MHC, coreceptors) using small molecules or biologic response modifiers

Abbreviations: APC, antigen-presenting cells HSP, heat shock protein; LNs, lymph nodes; TCR, T-cell receptor; MHC, major histocompatibility complex.

In this line, intra-LN immunization of patients with stage IV melanoma, with escalating doses of a plasmid expressing a tissue-specific antigen (tyrosinase), induced a heterogenous immune response—with only a few patients showing a robust immunity as assessed by tetramer staining (42). However, two interesting conclusions were drawn from this phase I clinical trial: First, despite some previous preclinical reports anticipating potential NF-kB-mediated toxic effects of plasmid, tolerability was excellent even at doses in excess of 1 mg. Secondly, there was a clear correlation between the clinical outlook (time to progression, time to death) and the immune response to tyrosinase (42). The latter implies either one of the following possibilities: (1) induction or amplification of immunity against this antigen results in an immune response that curbs the tumor progression or (2) an indirect correlation between immune responsiveness and the clinical outlook, possibly via immune mechanisms targeting other antigens that are not necessarily deployed by the plasmid.

One of the hallmarks of DNA immunization is the apparently excellent immune profile, encompassing T1 cells able to produce IFN-γ and other proinflammatory or effector cytokines, spanning both MHC class II– and class I–restricted subpopulations. The discovery, during the last decade, of a new class of immune-stimulating motifs in the form of unmethylated CpG palindromes (68) revolutionized the field of, and promoted interest in developing, synthetic CpG-based adjuvants as a counterpart of more conventional vaccines (69). The elucidation of a pattern recognition receptor (PRR) (TLR9) for unmethylated CpG motifs offered insight into the biologic role of this innate immune pathway, as a central mechanism of protection against important intracellular pathogens (70). Upon engagement of TLR9 and depending on the exact sequence of the palindrome, innate immune cells such as plasmacytoid DCs and other cell subsets rapidly produce IFN-α, IL-12, and additional T1-inducing mediators, via a MyD88/NF-kB signal transduction pathway (71). Hence, in the commonly referred model, it is believed that the T1-biasing adjuvant activity of plasmid vaccines encompassing unmethylated CpG motifs is due to the effect on innate immune cells via TLR9. However, unexpectedly, it was more recently shown that TLR9 knockout mice were still capable of generating T1 responses and IgG2a antibodies subsequent to DNA vaccination encompassing microbial antigens, challenging the previously proposed key role of TLR9 and leaving the door open for additional pathways of innate immune stimulation and/or mechanisms of induction of T1 response that are TLR independent (72).

In line with the numerous potential limiting factors downstream of APC transfection (Fig. 1), from antigen expression to a status of relative immune tolerance to self-antigens, it is imperative that those hurdles can be overcome without inserting additional, optimized CpG motifs. For example, while mRNA-based vaccination may circumvent the poor expression of plasmid in context of DNA vaccination (73), the adjuvant qualities of mRNA may be relatively reduced or at least modified relative to those of bacterial plasmids, unless ex vivo manipulation and activation of APCs is employed (74). On the other hand, however, it is not clear whether plasmid-borne CpG motifs indirectly interfere with transgene expression via innate immune stimulation (75).

CONCLUSIONS

In conclusion, numerous preclinical and subsequent clinical studies showed that plasmid vectors are able to induce immune responses; however, in many circumstances, such responses fall short of the magnitude required for protection against disease (in case of prophylactic vaccines), or disease suppression (in case of active immunotherapeutics). To summarize, the efficacy of current DNA vaccine vectors is still significantly reduced compared to that of viral vectors, in inducing a primary immune response. In contrast, the profile of the immune response elicited by DNA vaccines encompasses T1 cells (MHC class I– and/or class II–restricted, depending on the antigen expressed), and the subsequent immune memory seems to be long lived. Current clinical trials encompassing plasmid priming followed by boosting with heterologous vectors are aimed at addressing the important question, whether memory T cells elicited by DNA immunization can be effectively amplified in primates and turned into effector cells in prophylactic and therapeutic setting. More novel approaches targeting tissues rich in APCs may allow optimal utilization of nonviral-based vectors (such as peptides or recombinant proteins) as boosters. Nevertheless, especially in a therapeutic setting, troubleshooting the magnitude of immune response alone may not offer a complete solution, because of the multiplicity of the rate-limiting steps that are intrinsically linked to, or independent of, DNA immunization process. Only a systematic analysis and integrated approach relative to these limiting factors presented in this review—and others yet to be identified—would allow optimal utilization of DNA immunization concept in the clinic.

REFERENCES

1. Sedegah M, Hedstrom R, Hobart P, et al. Protection against malaria by immunization with plasmid DNA encoding circumsporozoite protein. Proc Natl Acad Sci U S A 1994; 91:9866–9870.
2. Ulmer JB, Donnelly JJ, Parker SE, et al. Heterologous protection against influenza by injection of DNA encoding a viral protein. Science 1993; 259:1745–1749.
3. Davis HL, Michel ML, Whalen RG. DNA-based immunization induces continuous secretion of hepatitis B surface antigen and high levels of circulating antibody. Hum Mol Genet 1993; 2:1847–1851.
4. Conry RM, LoBuglio AF, Kantor J, et al. Immune response to a carcinoembryonic antigen polynucleotide vaccine. Cancer Res 1994; 54:1164–1168.
5. Hawkins RE, Zhu D, Ovecka M, et al. Idiotypic vaccination against human B-cell lymphoma: rescue of variable region gene sequences from biopsy material for assembly as single-chain Fv personal vaccines. Blood 1994; 83:3279–3288.

6. Ciernik IF, Berzofsky JA, Carbone AP. Induction of cytotoxic T lymphocytes and antitumor immunity with DNA vaccines expressing single T cell epitopes. J Immunol 1996; 156:2369–2375.

7. Spellerberg MB, Zhu D, Thompsett A, et al. DNA vaccines against lymphoma: promotion of antiidiotypic antibody responses induced by single chain Fv genes by fusion to tetanus toxin fragment C. J Immunol 1997; 159:1885–1892.

8. Hsu CH, Chua KY, Tao MH, et al. Immunoprophylaxis of allergen-induced immunoglobulin E synthesis and airway hyperresponsiveness in vivo by genetic immunization. Nat Med 1996; 2:540–544.

9. Wildbaum G, Nahir MA, Karin N. Beneficial autoimmunity to proinflammatory mediators restrains the consequences of self-destructive immunity. Immunity 2003; 19:679–688.

10. Youssef S, Maor G, Wildbaum G, et al. C-C chemokine-encoding DNA vaccines enhance breakdown of tolerance to their gene products and treat ongoing adjuvant arthritis. J Clin Invest 2000; 106:361–371.

11. Liu MA, McClements W, Ulmer JB, et al. Immunization of non-human primates with DNA vaccines. Vaccine 1997; 15:909–912.

12. Leitner WW. Myth, menace or medical blessing? The clinical potential and problems of genetic vaccines. Expert Opin Biol Ther 2003; 3(1):1–4.

13. Barnett S, Otten SG, Srivastava I, et al. Enhanced DNA prime-protein boost vaccines induce potent immune responses against HIV-1. In Retroviruses of Human AIDS and Related Animal Diseases, XIII Cent Gardes Symposium. New York: Elsevier, 2003:145–153.

14. Cherpelis S, Shrivastava I, Gettie A, et al. DNA vaccination with the human immunodeficiency virus type 1 SF162ΔV2 envelope elicits immune responses that offer partial protection from simian/human immunodeficiency virus infection to CD8$^+$ T-cell-depleted rhesus macaques. J Virol 2001; 75:1547–1550.

15. Robinson HL, Montefiori DC, Johnson RP, et al. Neutralizing antibody-independent containment of immunodeficiency virus challenges by DNA priming and recombinant pox virus booster immunizations. Nat Med 1999; 5:526–534.

16. Li S, Rodrigues M, Rodriguez D, et al. Priming with recombinant influenza virus followed by administration of recombinant vaccinia virus induces CD8$^+$ T-cell-mediated protective immunity against malaria. Proc Natl Acad Sci USA 1993; 90:5214–5218.

17. Pardoll D. Does the immune system see tumors as foreign or self? Annu Rev Immunol 2003; 21:807–839.

18. Danko I, Williams P, Herweijer H, et al. High expression of naked plasmid DNA in muscles of young rodents. Hum Mol Genet 1997; 6:1435–1443.

19. Corr M, Lee DJ, Carson DA, et al. Gene vaccination with naked plasmid DNA: mechanism of CTL priming. J Exp Med 1996; 184:1555–1560.

20. Corr M, von Damm A, Lee DJ, et al. In vivo priming by DNA injection occurs predominantly by antigen transfer. J Immunol 1999; 163:4721–4727.

21. Klinman DM, Sechler G, Conover J, et al. Contribution of cells at the site of DNA vaccination to the generation of antigen specific immunity and memory. J Immunol 1998; 158:3635–3639.

22. Ulmer JB, Deck RR, DeWitt CM, et al. Expression of a viral protein by muscle cells in vivo induces protective cell-mediated immunity. Vaccine 1997; 15:839–845.

23. Fu TM, Ulmer JB, Caulfield MJ, et al. Priming of cytotoxic T lymphocytes by DNA vaccines: requirement for professional antigen presenting cells and evidence for antigen transfer from myocytes. Mol Med 1997; 3:362–371.

24. Spetz AL, Sorensen AS, Walther-Jallow L, et al. Induction of HIV-1-specific immunity after vaccination with apoptotic HIV-1/murine leukemia virus-infected cells. J Immunol 2002; 169:5771–5779.

25. Srivastava P. Interaction of heat shock proteins with peptides and antigen presenting cells: chaperoning of the innate and adaptive immune responses. Annu Rev Immunol 2002; 20:395–425.

26. Locher CP, Witt SA, Ashlock BM, et al. Enhancement of antibody responses to an HIV-2 DNA envelope vaccine using an expression vector containing a constitutive transport element. DNA Cell Biol 2002; 21:581–586.

27. Bot A, Stan AC, Inaba K, et al. Dendritic cells at a DNA vaccination site express the encoded influenza nucleoprotein and prime MHC class I-restricted cytolytic lymphocytes upon adoptive transfer. Int Immunol 2000; 12:825–832.

28. Dean DA, Dean BS, Muller S, et al. Sequence requirements for plasmid nuclear import. Exp Cell Res 1999; 253:713–722.

29. Porgador A, Irvine KR, Iwasaki A, et al. Predominant role for directly transfected dendritic cells in antigen presentation to CD8+ T cells after gene gun immunization. J Exp Med 1998; 188:1075–1082.

30. Barry MA, Johnston SA. Biological features of genetic immunization. Vaccine 1997; 15:788–791.

31. Condon C, Watkins SC, Celluzzi CM, et al. DNA-based immunization by in vivo transfection of dendritic cells. Nat Med 1996; 2:1122–1128.

32. Haddad D, Ramprakash J, Sedegah M, et al. Plasmid vaccine expressing granulocyte-macrophage colony-stimulating factor attracts infiltrates including immature dendritic cells into injected muscles. J Immunol 2000; 65:3772–3781.

33. Bins AD, Jorritsma A, Wolkers MC, et al. A rapid and potent DNA vaccination strategy defined by in vivo monitoring of antigen expression. Nat Med 2005; 11: 899–904.

34. Manam SB, Ledwith J, Barnum AB, et al. Plasmid DNA vaccines: tissue distribution and effects of DNA sequence, adjuvants and delivery method on integration into host DNA. Intervirology 2000; 43:273–281.

35. Denis-Mize KS, Dupuis M, MacKichan ML, et al. Plasmid DNA adsorbed onto cationic microparticles mediates target gene expression and antigen presentation by dendritic cells. Gene Ther 2000; 7:2105–2112.

36. Dupuis M, Denis-Mize MK, Woo C, et al. Distribution of DNA vaccines determines their immunogenicity after intramuscular injection in mice. J Immunol 2000; 165:2850–2858.

37. Maloy KL, Erdmann I, Basch V, et al. Intralymphatic immunization enhances DNA vaccination. Proc Natl Acad Sci USA 2001; 98:3299–3303.

38. Carcaboso AM, Hernández RM, Igartua M, et al. Enhancing immunogenicity and reducing dose of microparticulated synthetic vaccines: single intradermal administration. Pharm Res 2004; 21:121–126.

39. Velders MP, Weijzen S, Eiben GL. Defined flanking spacers and enhanced proteolysis is essential for eradication of established tumors by an epitope string DNA vaccine. J Immunol 2001; 166:5366–5373.

40. Moorthy VS, Imoukhuede EB, Keating S, et al. Phase 1 evaluation of 3 highly immunogenic prime-boost regimens, including a 12-month rebooting vaccination, for malaria vaccination in Gambian men. J Infect Dis 2004; 189:2213–2219.

41. Goonetilleke N, Moore S, Dally L, et al. Induction of multifunctional human immunodeficiency virus type 1 (HIV-1)-specific T cells capable of proliferation in healthy subjects by using a prime-boost regimen of DNA- and modified vaccinia virus Ankara-vectored vaccines expressing HIV-1 Gag coupled to CD8$^+$ T-cell epitopes. J Virol 2006; 80:4717–4728.

42. Tagawa ST, Lee P, Snively J, et al. Phase I study of intranodal delivery of a plasmid DNA vaccine for patients with Stage IV melanoma. Cancer 2003; 98:144–154.

43. Szmuness W, Stevens CE, Zang EA, et al. A controlled clinical trial of the efficacy of the hepatitis B vaccine (Heptavax B): a final report hepatology 1981; 1:377–385.

44. Beasley RP, Hwang LY, Lan CC, et al. Prevention of perinatally transmitted hepatitis B virus infections with hepatitis B immune globulin and hepatitis B vaccine. Lancet 1983; ii:1099–1102.

45. Liu MA, Ulmer JB. Human clinical trials of plasmid DNA vaccines. Adv Genet 2005; 55:25–40.

46. Mwau M, Cebere I, Sutton J, et al. A human immunodeficiency virus 1 (HIV-1) clade A vaccine in clinical trials: stimulation of HIV-specific T-cell responses by DNA and recombinant modified vaccinia virus Ankara (MVA) vaccines in humans. J Gen Virol 2004; 85:911–919.

47. Russell ND, Graham BS, Keefer MC, et al. Phase 2 study of an HIV-1 canarypox vaccine (vCP1452) alone and in combination with rgp120: negative results fail to trigger a phase 3 correlates trial. J Acquir Immune Defic Syndr 2007; 44:203–212.

48. McConkey SJ, Reece WH, Moorthy VS, et al. Enhanced T-cell immunogenicity of plasmid DNA vaccines boosted by recombinant modified vaccinia virus Ankara in humans. Nat Med 2003; 9:729–735.

49. Jager E, Karbach J, Gnjatic S, et al. Recombinant vaccinia/fowlpox NY-ESO-1 vaccines induce both humoral and cellular NY-ESO-1-specific immune responses in cancer patients. Proc Natl Acad Sci U S A 2006; 103:14453–14458.

50. Smith CL, Dunbar PR, Mirza F, et al. Recombinant modified vaccinia Ankara primes functionally activated CTL specific for a melanoma tumor antigen epitope in melanoma patients with a high risk of disease recurrence. Int J Cance. 2005; 113:259–266.

51. Kaufman HL, Wang W, Manola J, et al. Phase II randomized study of vaccine treatment of advanced prostate cancer (E7897): a trial of the Eastern Cooperative Oncology Group. J Clin Oncol 2004; 22:2122–2132.

52. Marshall JL, Hoyer RJ, Toomey MA, et al. Phase I study in advanced cancer patients of a diversified prime-and-boost vaccination protocol using recombinant vaccinia virus and recombinant nonreplicating avipox virus to elicit anti-carcinoembryonic antigen immune responses. J Clin Oncol 2000; 18:3964–3973.

53. Kongkasuriyachai D, Bartels-Andrews L, Stowers A, et al. Potent immunogenicity of DNA vaccines encoding *Plasmodium vivax* transmission-blocking vaccine candidates Pvs25 and Pvs28-evaluation of homologous and heterologous antigen-delivery prime-boost strategy. Vaccine 2004; 22:3205–3213.

54. Tanghe A, D'Souza S, Rosseels V, et al. Improved immunogenicity and protective efficacy of a tuberculosis DNA vaccine encoding Ag85 by protein boosting. Infect Immun 2001; 69:3041–3047.

55. Letvin NL, Huang Y, Chakrabarti BK. Heterologous envelope immunogens contribute to AIDS vaccine protection in rhesus monkeys. J Virol 2004; 78:7490–7497.
56. Jones TR, Narum DL, Gozalo AS, et al. Protection of Aotus monkeys by *Plasmodium falciparum* EBA-175 region II DNA prime-protein boost immunization regimen. J Infect Dis 2001; 183:303–312.
57. Irvine KR, Chamberlain RS, Shulman EP, et al. Enhancing efficacy of recombinant anticancer vaccines with prime/boost regimens that use two different vectors. J Natl Cancer Inst 1997; 89:1595–1601.
58. Meng WS, Butterfield LH, Ribas A, et al. Alpha-fetoprotein-specific tumor immunity induced by plasmid prime-adenovirus boost genetic vaccination. Cancer Res 2001; 61:8782–8786.
59. Nemunaitis J, Meyers T, Senzer N, et al. Phase I trial of sequential administration of recombinant DNA and adenovirus expressing L523S protein in early stage non-small-cell lung cancer. Mol Ther 2006; 13:1185–1191.
60. Naftzger C, Takechi Y, Kohda H, et al. Immune response to a differentiation antigen induced by altered antigen: a study of tumor rejection and autoimmunity. Proc Natl Acad Sci USA 1996; 93:14809–14814.
61. Weber LW, Bowne WB, Wolchok JD, et al. Tumor immunity and autoimmunity induced by immunization with homologous DNA. J Clin Invest 1998; 102:1258–1264.
62. Slovin S, Gregor P, Wolchok J, et al. A xenogeneic PSMA DNA vaccine for patients with non-castrate metastatic and castrate metastatic prostate cancer–A phase I trial of proof of principle. 43rd Annual Meeting of American Society of Clinical Oncology, Chicago, IL, June 1–5, 2007.
63. Wolchok JD, Gallardo H, Perales M, et al. Safety and immunogenicity of tyrosinase DNA vaccines in patients with melanoma. 43rd Annual Meeting of American Society of Clinical Oncology, Chicago, IL, June 1–5, 2007.
64. Foldvari M, Babiuk S, Badea I, et al. DNA delivery for vaccination and therapeutics through the skin. Curr Drug Deliv 2006; 3:17–28.
65. Buchan S, Grønevik E, Mathiesen I, et al. Electroporation as a "prime/boost" strategy for naked DNA vaccination against a tumor antigen. J Immunol 2005; 174: 6293–6298.
66. Johansen P, Haffner AC, Koch F, et al. Direct intralymphatic injection of peptide vaccines enhances immunogenicity. Eur J Immunol 2005; 35:568–574.
67. Pascolo S, Bervas N, Ure J, et al. HLA A2.1-restricted education and cytolytic activity of CD8+ T lymphocytes from beta2 microglobulin HLA A2.1 monochain transgenic H-2Db beta2m double knockout mice. J Exp Med 1997; 185:2043–2051.
68. Wagner H. Bacterial CpG DNA activates immune cells to signal infectious danger. Adv Immunol 1999; 73:329–368.
69. Klinman DM. Adjuvant activity of CpG oligodeoxynucleotides. Int Rev Immunol 2006; 25:135–154.
70. Hemmi H, Takeuchi O, Kawai T, et al. A toll-like receptor recognizes bacterial DNA. Nature 2000; 408:740–745.
71. Wagner H. The immunobiology of the TLR9 subfamily. Trends Immunol 2004; 25:381–386.
72. Hemmi H, Kaisho T, Takeda K, et al. The roles of toll-like receptor 9, MyD88, and DNA-dependent protein kinase catalytic subunit in the effects of two distinct CpG DNAs on dendritic cell subsets. J Immunol 2003; 170:3059–3064.

73. Grunebach F, Muller MR, Nencioni A, et al. Delivery of tumor-derived RNA for the induction of cytotoxic T-lymphocytes. Gene Ther 2003; 10:367–374.
74. Bontkes HJ, Kramer D, Ruizendaal JJ, et al. Dendritic cells transfected with interleukin-12 and tumor-associated antigen messenger RNA induce high avidity cytotoxic T cells. Gene Ther 2007; 14:366–375.
75. Payette PJ, Ma X, Weeratna RD, et al. Testing of CpG-optimized protein and DNA vaccines against the hepatitis B virus in chimpanzees for immunogenicity and protection from challenge. Intervirology 2006; 49:144–151.

Bidirectional Bedside Lab Bench Processes and Flexible Trial Design as a Means to Expedite the Development of Novel Immunotherapeutics

Adrian Bot

MannKind Corporation, Valencia, California, U.S.A.

Mihail Obrocea

MannKind Corporation, Paramus, New Jersey, U.S.A.

INTRODUCTION

In this chapter, we propose the revision of several paradigms defining research and development (R&D) processes in support of investigational drugs. The emergence of many investigational molecular targeted therapies stimulated by an unprecedented progress in the genomics arena raised new challenges in drug development. In the era of molecular medicine, a major objective of modern translational research is to identify the target with the most optimal clinical opportunity. This is noticeably illustrated in the case of "first in class" investigational drugs without existing benchmark in terms of approved products. Using innovative cancer vaccines as a study case, we illustrate several key revisions of the drug development process aimed to expedite and optimize the drug development decisional stages. These proposed key modifications are (1) revising the role of preclinical models, (2) implementing biomarker-guided processes during early exploration, and (3) considering novel, adaptive trial designs to direct clinical development in a more optimal fashion.

"CANCER VACCINES": KEY ELEMENTS AND CHALLENGES

"Cancer vaccines" or active immunotherapeutics encompass defined antigens, analogues, or fragments, which are in fact molecular targeted agents. Immune cells such as Th or Tc cells or antibodies elicited by the vaccine are aimed to recognize specific molecules expressed by cancer cells or within the tumor environment. The indirect mechanism of action (MOA) is a distinctive property of cancer vaccines compared to other molecular targeted therapies. Particularly, while monoclonal antibodies or tyrosine kinase inhibitors act directly on receptors and affect cell viability or signal transduction pathways, vaccines relay on their capability to induce immune mediators that in turn act on the target (Fig. 1). This has far-reaching implications in the R&D of such investigational agents and presents a set of unique challenges that distinguish this class of drug candidates from all others. In addition, there is no current benchmark in terms of approved cancer vaccine in the United States, increasing the complexity, risk, and heterogeneity of the current development strategies. The difficulty associated with establishing appropriate preclinical models along with a relative complex MOA hinders their predictability. By using preclinical models more often, it has been easier to predict whether a vaccine induced immunity in humans, as opposed to whether an immune response translated into clinical outcome. Unfortunately, this limitation along with the sub-optimal clinical efficacy of investigational cancer vaccines evaluated in the past precluded the definition of reliable pharmacodynamic (PD) markers and surrogate endpoints that are key to guide and accelerate the development process. Moreover, the different safety profiles from that of more conventional classes of drugs and the considerable heterogeneity in terms of technology platforms—from highly personalized, cell based, to microbial vectors and synthetic, nonreplicating molecules—are distinct features of investigational cancer vaccines posing significant challenges in

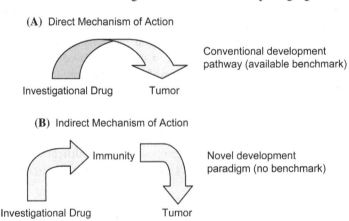

Figure 1 Challenges posed by development of cancer vaccines as largely related to the indirect nature of their mechanism of action.

both preclinical toxicology strategy and the design and identification of end points in clinical trials. Altogether, these characteristics define critical gaps in the development of cancer vaccines: (1) between preclinical development and clinical exploration due to the complexity of MOA and limited predictability of most preclinical models and (2) between early- and late-stage clinical development due to the scarcity of PD and surrogate end points to guide to development process.

REDESIGNED R&D STRATEGY IN SUPPORT OF "CANCER VACCINES"

To meet these challenges and aim for an appropriate testing of proof of concept, as well as identification of optimal candidates for randomized proof of concept trials, one needs to consider different approaches of development for active immunotherapies in cancer versus drugs with a more direct MOA.

First and foremost, to bridge the gap between preclinical exploration and clinical evaluation, we need to abandon the classical linear development process and instead factor in the complementary value of data gathered in preclinical and clinical models in support of selecting the right lead candidate. This selection will have a profound outcome on the development process, for example, from design, optimization, and preclinical exploration to Investigational new drug application (IND)-enabling studies followed by proof of concept trials and finally, confirmatory phase 3 trials. Essentially, this will translate into a two-way approach—bench to bed and reverse—aiming to ensure optimization of the therapeutic candidate (composition, regimen, tumor type, and indication) prior to initiating larger randomized trials (Fig. 2).

(**A**) Linear development process

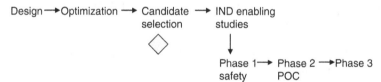

(**B**) Bench to bedside and reverse

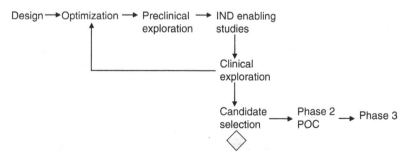

Figure 2 A comparison between linear and cyclical development paths of second generation (**A**) or first in class (**B**) investigational compounds.

Another key aspect of the new paradigm is the implementation of a bio-marker-guided approach as early as possible during the development process in order to optimize and expedite proof of concept evaluation in a manner that increases the likelihood of success and reduces the size of clinical trials. The concept of "stratified medicine" or "theranostic approach" implies, in essence, definition and use of biomarkers as inclusion/exclusion criteria to direct the evaluation of the investigational drug in patients that have highest likelihood of clinical response.

Another aspect, resulting from the complexity of the MOA and insufficiency of preclinical models, is the re-evaluation of the clinical response. While in more conventional situations—such as those corresponding to investigational drugs that influence tumoral cells directly—the predictable nature of in vitro and preclinical modeling is established and accepted to a higher extent. In the case of active immunotherapies, the value of preclinical evaluation may consist rather in exploring the limits of the technology that will impact the design of clinical studies, thus having a higher likelihood of being informative or meeting preset success criteria.

Finally, in light of the early development stage of most cancer active immunotherapeutics currently, it is key to leverage emerging proof of concept data in clinic generated with more mature technology platforms into novel approaches. More specifically, significant steps were undertaken in demonstrating proof of concept in clinic with cell-based vaccines (e.g., autologous dendritic cells (DCs) expressing target antigens or GM-CSF producing allogeneic tumor cells), leading the way to late-stage development. While these technology platforms have certain drawbacks, such as reliance on patient's cells or collection of poorly defined cellular antigens, information from clinic on their performance is important for the development of newer "off-the-shelf" and synthetic molecules, allowing a more expedite development process with increased chances of success.

In the next paragraph, we focus on several factors outlined above (such as the significance of preclinical and clinical exploration), the fundamental role of biomarkers, and finally, exemplification with an investigational approach in early clinical development.

REVISING THE ROLE OF PRECLINICAL STUDIES

Cancer immunotherapeutic approaches require quite cumbersome preclinical modeling due to the inherent complexity of the MOA of therapeutic platforms under development. Useful models—with capability to predict the PD profile of an investigational drug—need to meet key criteria; nevertheless, due to intrinsic differences of immune responsiveness and antigenic makeup between species (Fig. 3), it has been very difficult if not impossible to envision a model equivalent to, for example, the xenograft models used in preclinical pharmacology in support of development of small molecules. One of the most illustrious examples

Similarities and differences between preclinical models and clinical setting

Similarities	Generally similar immune regulation mechanisms Immunogenicity is generally translatable (yes/no)
Differences	Antigen identity and sequence differs Magnitude and profile of immune response may differ Translation of immune response into tumor response Overall status of immune responsiveness (pretreatment) Responsiveness to biological response modifiers

Figure 3 The gap between preclinical models and clinical setting for cancer vaccine development.

of technology facing significant hurdles in translation from preclinical to clinical stage results from the fact that cancer vaccines are based on defined antigens. Such vaccine candidates encompass a variety of vectors (polypeptides, cells, microbes, recombinant DNA), immunological information (epitopes) corresponding to the antigenic makeup of tumor cells, with the aim to instruct one's cells to recognize and react against the malignant process. Despite the fact that it has been recognized that the immune systems in rodent and humans, for example, operate in quite similar fashion, the sequence of the overwhelming majority of defined epitopes within tumor antigens of interest is not identical between mouse and man. Even if new tools became available, such as HLA transgenic mice, overcoming significant differences in the T-cell repertoire in mouse and man, due to differential MHC restriction, the distinct antigen sequence poses formidable hurdles in face of deploying animal models for predicting the magnitude and quality of immune response to human epitopes. Most significantly, a human epitope translated into an investigational drug that encompasses even one amino acid difference at the TCR-engaging site relative to the rodent version is recognized as "nonself" by the immune system. This results into a more potent response that one would otherwise occur in the desired, ultimate setting. An overestimation of pharmacological potency of antigen-based vaccines by using preclinical modeling may occur, in addition, when differences between mouse and human sequences affect primary MHC anchor residues, rendering, for example, the mouse version irrelevant and the human one "nonself." Thus, while there is some agreement that animal models can be employed to compare various methods of immunization and generally predict immunogenicity of an investigational compound in clinic, considerations outlined above and others (such as dosing) preclude accurate translation of magnitude and profile of immune response from preclinical models to clinical setting.

Another aspect that has been even more difficult to model and translate to clinic was the impact of immune response on tumor regression or clinical outcome in general due to the fact that transplantable tumors are highly artificial. Models involving spontaneously arising tumors were developed—yet the nature of therapeutic targets in preclinical setting, with some exceptions, limited their value in relation to exploration of humanized investigational drugs. Overall, it was not yet possible to reproduce in a preclinical model the target expression environment within a human tumor—one reason was the complexity and scarcity of reliable information regarding the latter.

A distinct feature that has been notoriously difficult to reproduce in pre-clinical setting has been the strict status of the immune system and immune repertoire from patients treated with multiple standard therapies (such as radio and/or chemotherapy). Since the MOA of active immunotherapies requires immune competence, this represents a major parameter. In fact, attempts to explore this question resulted in tantalizing observations consisting in additive or even synergistic effects between select chemotherapies (cyclophosphamide, paclitaxel, doxorubicin, cisplatin) and vaccination. Beyond the interesting sci-entific explanation having to do with a T-cell repertoire conditioning or inter-ference with immune "breaks," or the practical implications on designing innovative combination approaches in clinic, a major criticism remains: The effect of chemotherapies on immune system seems to be species specific so thorough clinical exploration is needed to elucidate whether these observations truly translate to man.

Finally, a major difference between preclinical and clinical setting—that limits the translation of findings from the former to the latter—is the species-specific recognition and response to "biological response modifiers" or adjuvants in general. To be active, cancer vaccines rely on delivery of not only immu-nological information such as epitopes but, at the same time, of motifs or molecules that instruct the immune system to mount a response of a certain magnitude and profile, most often by influencing the innate immunity. Most recently, such molecules have been described as TLR ligands (CpG motifs binding to TLR9; ds or ssRNA binding to TLR3, 7, and/or 8; LPS analogues binding to TLR4; and even small molecules binding to TLR7 such as Imiqui-mode®) that exert their function by activating receptor-positive DCs, NK cells, or other cells of the immune system. Since receptor distribution on cell subsets, the relative function of different subsets, and the fine specificity of receptors vary from species to species, it is not unexpected that, for example, the TLR9 ligands CpG motifs have a different optimal structure in relation to an effective innate immune stimulation in mouse and human. Therefore, preclinical modeling may not be entirely predictive relative to immune-stimulating properties of vaccine excipients.

Altogether, these issues suffice to raise a fundamental question that is highly applicable to the preclinical modeling of active immunotherapies in cancer, but to a lesser extent to other therapeutic strategies relying on more direct mechanisms of action. Namely, one needs to acknowledge that preclinical evaluation of an investigational drug, like a cancer vaccine aimed to treat a human disease, is intrinsically limited in its predictable value. Paradoxically, preclinical modeling using humanized investigational drugs may be even more artificial in certain cases, as opposed to using model reagents. For example, asking key questions on whether an immunization approach can "break toler-ance" against a self-tumor antigen. Thus, it seems that the value of preclinical modeling in support of active immunotherapies needs to be revised. We propose that instead of being used as a framework to test the pharmacology of humanized investigational drugs and bridge mechanically the discovery/optimization with the clinical stage, preclinical exploration's mission in the case of cancer vaccines is to clarify key questions on their applicability and optimization strategy prior to initiating and in conjunction with clinical evaluation. If we recognize that every preclinical model or setting is defined by a set of parameters (e.g., the nature and potency of immunization approach, the match between the vaccine composition and target antigen on the tumor, and the level of expression of the target antigen and host's immune competency), then preclinical exploration using highly experimental reagents would be capable of defining the limits and opportunities associated with a therapeutic approach. The impact on clinical strategy is vast since that way we direct the subsequent clinical exploration in a manner that would maximize the likelihood of success and minimize the risk.

To exemplify, if we idealize the parameters enumerated above (use of an extremely potent immunization approach that leverages response against a "nonself" antigen, use of a transplantable tumor that is highly immunogenic in animals that are immune competent), the resulting experimental setting would allow us to answer a key question: Is cancer vaccination in its most potent version effective enough to trigger objective tumor regression in bulky disease setting? This is not a trivial question since it has been recently showed that while adoptive T-cell therapy with large number of activated effector cells resulted in tumor regression in man, previous vaccines failed to show that—on the other hand their modest immunogenicity has been a great confounding factor. As shown in Figure 4, summarizing the conclusion from literature, it seems that

Impact on:	Experimental approach	Success	Clinical relevance
Prevention of tumor formation	Immunization first	+	N/A
Circulating tumor cells	In vivo cytotoxicity	+	Adjuvant
Micrometastases	Immunize in MRD setting	+ / -	Adjuvant
Limited lesions	Immunize in min tumor setting	+ / -	Consolidation
Bulky tumors	Immunize in bulky tumor setting	+ / - -	Refractory

Figure 4 Relevance of preclinical modeling to define optimal clinical indications for cancer vaccines.

preclinical modeling is actually capable to provide key answers to this question and firmly define the limitations of applicability to cancer vaccines. Most attempts to immunize in a prophylactic setting against tumor challenge or spontaneous tumor formation were met by success, irrespective of the platform technology used—a strong argument in support of the fact that the needed threshold in terms of magnitude of immune response or stringency related to the profile of immunity were low. That is actually the strongest criticism against overinterpreting data sets from clinical studies generated across different vaccine platforms—many of them proved subsequently to be quite suboptimal—in an established tumor setting. Whether cancer vaccines "work" or "do not work" is a question that is highly dependent on both the vaccine platform as well as the clinical setting in which they are tested. For example, data sets generated in preclinical models comprising limited solid tumor burden, with potent vaccination approaches, strongly suggest that immunization alone can be a quite effective means to objectively impact tumor progression. Unfortunately, immunization alone rarely achieves objective regression in a bulky tumor setting despite an optimal antigenic match between tumor and vaccine and a competent immune system. In contrast, achieving a strong systemic response may result in elimination of circulating tumor cells and obliteration of metastatic lesions. This is a key feature that may in fact impact survival by blocking disease spread or relapse, mainly responsible for serious morbidity and mortality in cancer. Altogether, this exemplifies how preclinical exploration sheds light on the limits of active immunotherapy or cancer vaccines: They are more likely to succeed in limited disease setting or minimal residual disease in indications such as adjuvant or consolidation therapy. Conversely, this along with mechanistic studies strongly suggested that in order for vaccination "to work" in a bulky or advance disease setting, one needs to contemplate more complex approaches that encompass the immunogen as well as compounds that interfere with various immune breaks limiting the activity of immune effector cells within tumors.

More recently, the conventional wisdom that chemotherapy unavoidably hampers active immunotherapy has been seriously challenged by numerous findings in idealized preclinical settings encompassing both autoimmunity and vaccination against tumor antigens. From a mechanistic standpoint, it became clear that the time window associated with recovery of the T-cell repertoire offers an opportunity to induce tolerance or conversely, repopulate the immune system with antigen-specific T cells by vaccination. Chemotherapies, novel small molecules, or biomolecules may positively affect the outcome of active immunotherapy at multiple levels (Fig. 5). All of that can be explored by employing preclinical models such as:

1. Amplifying the frequency of antigen-specific T cells by vaccination post-lymphodepletion carried out by chemotherapy (with or without myeloablation);

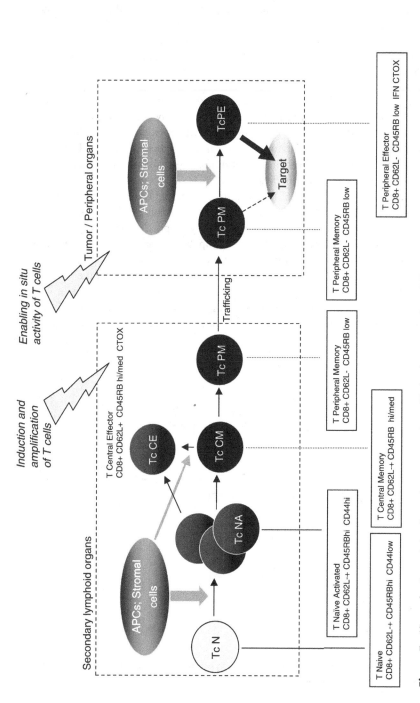

Figure 5 (*See color insert.*) A schematic representation of induction, expansion, differentiation, and migration of tumor antigen–specific T cells upon vaccination against tumor-associated antigens. *Abbreviations:* TcN, T cytotoxic naive; Tc NA, Tc naive activated; Tc CM, Tc central memory; Tc CE, Tc effectors; Tc PM, Tc peripheral memory; Tc PE, Tc peripheral effectors.

2. Inducting disease reduction or complete remission by chemotherapy prior to initiation of active immunotherapy, aimed to reduce the tumor burden and thus enable the overall activity of immunity; and

3. Interfering with checkpoints or immune breaks within tumor tissue, thus enabling the activity of effector T cells—for example, by interfering with T regulatory cells.

This concept is being currently evaluated in clinic as such or in various formats: nonmyeloablative transient lymphodepletion by cyclophosphamide and/ or fludarabine followed by vaccination (1), myeloablative chemoradiotherapy followed by autologous T-lymphocyte transfer, and vaccination plus IL-2 (2) or combination approaches of vaccines plus biological response modifiers such as anti-CTLA-4 monoclonal antibodies (3).

The differential activity of tumor antigen–specific T cells within lymphoid organs, peripheral organs bearing micrometastases versus larger tumors, can be readily analyzed in preclinical models with key impact on understanding the translation to clinic. For example, immunocompetent mice bearing large primary tumors and micrometastases mount immune responses upon vaccination against tumor-specific antigens to explore the impact of specific T cells on the viability of antigen-bearing target cells within large tumors, or systemically, an in vivo CFSE cytotoxic assay can be employed (Fig. 6). Control cells ("mock") and antigen-expressing cells ("targets") tagged with CFSE at a different intensity can

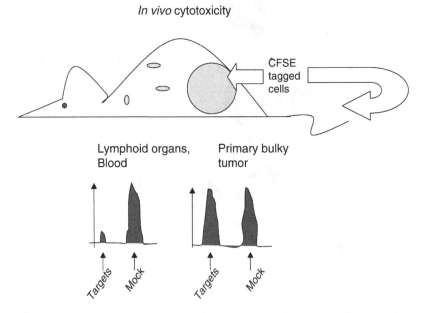

Figure 6 Schematic representation of a prototype study to assess the systemic versus local functionality of tumor-specific T cells.

be infused systemically and directly into the primary tumor. The relative removal of target cells can be assessed at various time points both within tumor and peripheral lymphoid or nonlymphoid organs containing metastatic tumor cells. An accumulating body of evidence supports the view that despite trafficking of tumor-specific T cells into the primary tumor, the specific activity within the tumor is limited in contrast to the optimal removal of antigenic target cells within peripheral lymphoid organs and blood (Fig. 6). Altogether, it appears that in a setting of immune competence, successful induction of tumor-specific immunity results in optimal systemic immune surveillance compatible with removal of M0/M1-circulating cells and micrometastatic foci without effectively interfering with tumor-cell viability within bulky tumor lesions.

Another key question related to optimal translation of investigational active immunotherapies is the duration and intensity of the immunization protocol; this question is relevant since only a minor fraction (1% or less) of the elicited tumor-specific T cells have the capability to produce proinflammatory or cytotoxic mediators upon contact with tumor cells. This supports the model in which most of the tumor-antigen-specific T cells elicited by active immunotherapy do not have an optimal functional avidity and indicate the need to improve on this parameter by deploying more advanced vaccination methods. Therefore, a key parameter to be followed—in addition to the magnitude of the immune response and its effector profile—is the functional avidity as expressed by the slope of the curve in Figure 7 (angle Ω, corresponding to the ratio between the variation of frequency of tumor-reactive cells and the variation of frequency of antigen-specific cells measured in condition of optimal restimulation of T cells with synthetic peptide).

The relationship between the immune response to vaccine and the immune modulating activity of the tumor process can be modeled as well to a certain extent; there are at least two scenarios from the standpoint of whether vaccine-elicited

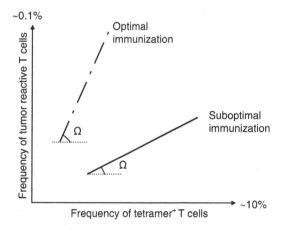

Figure 7 Definition functional avidity of tumor antigen–specific T cells.

immunity initiates or does not initiate a self-perpetuating response against the tumor. In the first scenario, tumor antigen–specific T cells induced or activated by the active immunotherapeutic regimen, traffic to the tumor site where they affect the viability of target tumor cells. Subsequently, antigens liberated by the tumor cells are internalized and processed by resident antigen-presenting cells (APCs) that migrate to regional lymph nodes where they successfully restimulate, amplify, or maintain the immune response to the immunizing antigen and even additional tumor-specific antigens. In this model, subsequent immunization to maintain a level of effector cells within tumor or lymphoid organs would not be necessary since the direct stimulating effect of the tumor is under the attack of vaccine-induced T cells. In the second model, while the vaccine is able to elicit a population of tumor antigen–specific T cells encompassing high-avidity T cells, tumor-derived antigen is not sufficient to maintain or amplify the immune response. This results in the model depicted in Figure 8, quite supported by experimental evidence. More specifically, repeat administration of antigen would be instrumental not only for eliciting a response with a maximum potential, but to maintain a subpopulation of high-avidity functional T cells with activity against tumor cells. In absence of continuing the immunization process, the tumor cells alone would be incapable to drive expansion and differentiation of memory T cells to effector cells, with serious consequences in terms of the

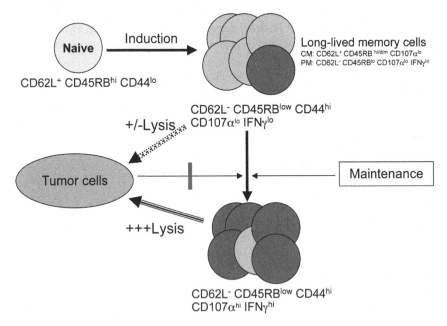

Figure 8 A schematic depiction of the functional, immunologic relationship between tumor antigens–specific T cells and tumor cells, with impact on design-improved immunotherapeutic approaches.

efficacy and vaccine-induced immune response. Thus, in essence, the induction of immune response would be aimed at eliciting central-memory (CM) T cells with a capability to further expand to peripheral memory (PM) and differentiate to peripheral effector (PE) cells, trafficking to the tumor site, and exerting antitumor cell activity inasmuch as there are T cells endowed with high functional avidity present. It is expected that host's immune homeostatic mechanisms together with tumor's environment result in exhaustion, apoptosis, and shrinkage of the self-tumor antigen–specific PE T-cell population. The subsequent immunization steps would be aimed to reelicit expansion and differentiation of PE cells from CM cells. Overall, repeat immunization would ensure reinduction of CM cells and differentiation of PE cells present in the system in an intermittent rather than continuous fashion. In addition, should there be induction of anticognate tumor antigen–specific T cells that promote a proinflammatory process, there is a possibility of "epitope spreading" that is mirrored by activation, expansion, and differentiation of T cells specific for other tumor antigens. Nevertheless, while the evidence in support of this phenomenon is quite limited (4), epitope spreading would be able to preempt—to a certain extent—immune escape mechanisms consisting in antigen loss.

Despite the difficulties associated with the translation of observations from preclinical models to clinic, preclinical exploration is still important to optimize and advance complex active immunotherapeutic approaches to clinic. Exploration of "idealized" models encompassing dominant antigens and powerful methods of immunization in immune-competent organisms shed light on the limits of active immunotherapy and pinpoint the nature of indications associated with least chance of success in the clinic. Conversely, preclinical exploration provides hints regarding the type of indications to be explored in clinic and the end points to be evaluated (Fig. 9):

1. Minimal residual disease, postdebulking using surgery or other means that do not induce a persisting immune suppression ("adjuvant" approach); clinical end points may be overall survival, progression-free survival, and time to relapse.
2. Limited but measurable disease (metastatic or isolated lesions), in a setting that may or may not follow standard therapy that partially reduced the tumor burden without inducing persisting immune suppression; clinical end points may be progression-free survival, overall survival, tumor regression, and/or time to progression (TTP).
3. Bulky disease (metastatic or isolated lesions), refractory to standard therapy alone or rapidly relapsing, in a setting where immune competence is preserved. In that case, while active immunotherapy alone is not expected to impact disease progression, there is a potential that carefully selected combination approaches result in clinical benefit (increased response rate manifested through partial tumor regression, disease

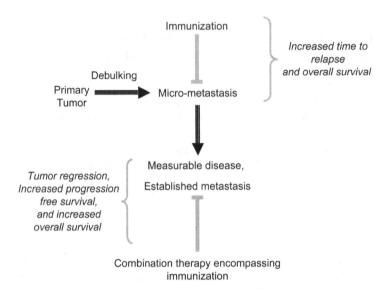

Figure 9 Defining the unmet clinical need vis-à-vis the potential of innovative immunotherapeutic approaches or cancer vaccines.

stabilization, increased TTP, overall survival, and/or quality of life). There is still a significant amount of work that needs to be carried out both in preclinical models and in clinic to define combination approaches with impact on tumor progression; several candidates tested are: cyclophosphamide, fludarabine, doxorubicine, paclitaxel, or biological response modifiers such as anti-CTLA4, anti-CD25, or anti-CD4 monoclonal antibodies.

BIOMARKER-GUIDED R&D

In support of several components of the development process, the hallmarks of the new molecular targeted therapies are biomarkers. Unfortunately, there is a significant heterogeneity of biomarkers, somewhat hampering the communication in this area. We depicted three general categories of biomarkers in Figure 10, based on the scientific significance, utility, and implication to the drug development process.

First, markers of disease, disease relapse, or progression are correlates of the pathologic process. Higher the disease burden, higher the level of such biomarkers or analytes. While there are very few sensitive and specific biomarkers in cancer, clusters of biomarkers as opposed to individual markers may be more reliable if they correlate with disease relapse or progression. In the context of cancer vaccines, such biomarkers may be key to identify individuals

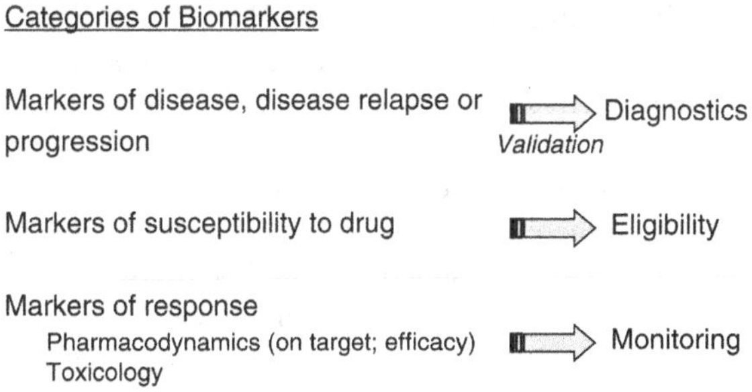

Categories of Biomarkers

Markers of disease, disease relapse or progression   ▥⟹ Diagnostics
Validation

Markers of susceptibility to drug   ▥⟹ Eligibility

Markers of response
   Pharmacodynamics (on target; efficacy)   ▥⟹ Monitoring
   Toxicology

Figure 10   The diversity of biomarkers and their usefulness.

that started to relapse or progress after standard therapy, while the process is not clinically evident yet (e.g., PSA- or CA-125-positive patients with no overt clinical disease). The reason is that cancer vaccines are more applicable to indications associated with limited disease burden or minimal residual disease; therefore, identifying patients in that earlier stage is of paramount importance. In addition, since the length of clinical trials is a limiting factor in the development of therapies for oncologic disorders, in a setting of limited disease, biomarkers that correlate and anticipate clinical progression are critical in providing timely data set that would support a rationale for a decisional process. Finally, patient stratification approaches based on biomarkers and applied to minimum residual disease post-standard therapy may result in identification and expedited evaluation of efficacy of investigational agents. There are quite several markers in this expanding category such as VEGF, CA-125, and PSA. If validated through clinical experimentation, such biomarkers—alone or as clusters—may become important diagnostics complementary to more conventional approaches. With the emerging maturation of various databases on biomarker expression in human normal tissues as well as diseased tissues or tumor archives resulting from worldwide omics efforts, there is an exciting possibility for target discovery based on biomarker database mining. Careful computer-based analysis of proteomics, transcriptomics, and genomics data may reveal entire signal transduction pathways with associated membrane receptors amenable to biomolecule targeting and downstream enzymes that can be targeted via conventional small molecule technologies.

A category of biomarkers of paramount importance for the development of new molecular targeted therapies is that of markers that predict responsiveness to an investigational drug. Since molecular pathogenesis and thus tumor susceptibility to drugs is quite heterogeneous, these biomarkers have a severalfold impact: First, they would outline a subpopulation of patients that would benefit the most from drug exposure; second, that would minimize unnecessary exposure of patients that are less likely to benefit from the drug. Overall, this would lead to more rapid, focused development of the drug by increasing therapeutic index, efficacy-to-noise ratio, diminishing the size of the clinical trials, and improving the odds that a specific investigational agent studied will gain market approval by the regulatory authorities. An obvious subcategory of biomarkers considered is that of target molecules themselves. If the target molecule is not expressed within the tumor tissue, irrespective of the MOA, the likelihood of clinical response is diminished should there be no significant "off target" effects. Well-known examples for such biomarkers in support of antibody-based treatment are Her-2/Neu expression or CD20 expression by tumor cells defining patients eligible for transtuzumab or rituximab treatment, respectively; but the paradigm spans other categories of molecular targeted therapies such as small molecules (bcr/abl in the case of imatinib, and EGFR polymorphism for gefitinib). It is not difficult to imagine that by not having a biomarker-based approach to stratify patients what would have been the fate of trastuzumab (Herceptin®) since the treatment is relevant to only ~ 35% of breast carcinoma patients that display upregulation of Her-2/Neu. Due to the indirect and complex MOA, the challenges faced by active immunotherapy in light of this are considerably more significant. It would be ideal to have appropriate reagents and methodologies to determine and quantify the targets in clinical setting since the target molecules in many cases are MHC-peptide complexes expressed by the tumor cells. Unfortunately, this field is not mature yet; nevertheless, there is exciting new research on a new generation of antibody-like molecules that directly recognize MHC-peptide complexes (5). In the absence of measuring the target molecules, the next best approach—used by several groups developing antigen-based cancer vaccines—is to measure by immunohistochemistry the target antigen and MHC class I expression. Due to the fact that antigen processing and presentation is heterogeneous and subject to a variety of immune escape phenomena, this is obviously only a surrogate for target (MHC-peptide) molecule expression. A difficult aspect related to using such biomarkers is the correlation of the pharmacological activity with their biomarkers' level of expression; in addition, the magnitude of the activity may depend to a high extent on the nature and potency of the investigational drug. Other approaches, for example, based on whole tumor lysates, allogeneic tumor cells or in general, not directed to a specific but a collection of antigens may not benefit from a target-related biomarker strategy. This increases considerably the risk throughout development. If we just consider the fact that a significant percentage of tumors show clear immune escape phenomena via MHC class I and/or TAP defects (between 20 and 50%), a lack of patient stratification based on target molecule expression may have drastic consequences in terms of reduction in response rate (even assuming an excellent pharmacological effect of the investigational drug). Conversely, use of such biomarker-based approaches to direct the testing of investigational agents in select populations—when afforded by the immunotherapeutic strategy—may have a negative impact on the number of patients treated in a specific disease setting. However this may ultimately result in an enhanced opportunity from medical and commercial standpoint due to a likely increased efficacy in clinic.

Requirements for translation of drug exposure into a clinical effect
•Factors X, Y, Z, etc

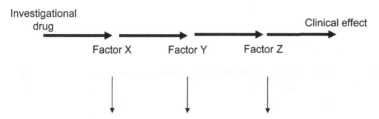

Key molecular features of MOA can be translated into biomarkers
predicting <u>diminished</u> likelihood of response

$$R_0 = N_r / N_t \implies R_\sigma = N_r / (N_t - N_{ne}) \implies R\sigma / R0 = N_t / (N_t - N_{ne})$$
Where R_0 is the rate of response without patient stratification, Nr is the number
of patients showing response; Nt is the total number of patients; $R\sigma$ is the rate of response when
stratification is carried out; N_{ne} is the number of non-eligible patients based on definitive
exclusion criteria resulting from MOA

Figure 11 Modeling the impact of biomarkers related to the mechanism of action, on the development of investigational drugs with complex (indirect) mechanism of action, such as cancer vaccines.

In face of the shear complexity of the MOA of all active immunotherapies in development, we propose a different strategy to define target patient populations; namely, by delineating ineligibility criteria based on thorough understanding of the MOA (Fig. 11). For example, in order for a cancer vaccine to have an impact on the tumor process, an immune response must be mounted— for example, specific cytotoxic T cells (CTLs) that must migrate to the tumor site overcome immune checkpoints within the tumor environment, recognize MHC class I complexes, and trigger optimal effector mechanisms that result in altering the viability of tumor cells. Even if we stay at this simplistic level, one realizes that if any of the following criteria are not met, then the likelihood of a clinical effect elicited by the vaccine therapy would be near zero due to the following issues: (1) the patient's immune system may be suppressed; (2) the patient does not carry the right MHC allele in the case of epitope-based immunization; (3) the patient's tumor cells do not express MHC class I; (4) the patient's tumor cells do not express the target antigens; and/or (5) the patient's tumor is a strongly immune suppressive environment (no lymphocytes). Thus, parameters that define the situations above become biomarkers that can be used to screen patients eligible for the treatment; this approach to identify failure-linked biomarkers is considerably easier than defining biomarkers that positively predict clinical response during early development stages. Mathematically, use of multiple failure-prediction biomarkers in support of this approach (patient screening) would be as beneficial yet more easier compared to defining response-prediction biomarkers. For example, in the case of a hypothetical epitope targeted approach as an investigational cancer vaccine, lack of target antigen expression within tumor (let us assume that it represents 40% of the patient population), and of the right HLA type (in the case of A2 corresponding at least to about 50% of patient population), the new rate of response—according to the formula shown in Fig. 11 inset—would be fivefold higher upon biomarker-based patient stratification in an intent to treat setting and assuming efficacy of the investigational compound. This approach could make the difference between a successful and an unsuccessful investigational drug in early development phase when trial sizes are small and companies are seeking to make swift go/no-go decisions and conserve resources. In aggregate, this category of biomarkers may likely translate into eligibility criteria that are part of the design of exploratory proof of mechanism and proof of concept trials having a critical role in defining the development strategy.

The third category of biomarkers of value in assisting investigational drug development relevant to molecular targeted approaches such as cancer vaccines are markers of pharmacological and toxicological effects. The MOA of cancer vaccines is indirect and in the absence of clear indications to pursue in large pivotal trials, there needs to be a strategy to advance investigational drugs more rapidly through early clinical development and reach go/no-go decisions based on rationale, sound data set, and best possible indications to pursue. Therefore, collecting comprehensive information on the activity of the drug candidate during exploratory preclinical studies and trials is of paramount importance. The Figure 12 depicts this principle that is equally applicable—for investigational

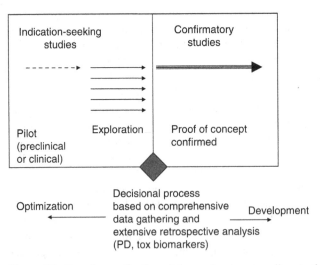

Figure 12 Iterative application of the exploratory paradigm to the preclinical as well as the clinical stage in development of cancer vaccines and, in general, of molecular targeted approaches.

targeted therapies such as active immunotherapies—to both the preclinical and clinical phases of drug development. The aim of exploration is twofold: first, demonstrating proof of concept and outlining appropriate end points and second, defining the most optimal settings or indications to take an investigational drug in confirmatory studies. One should also not forget that "off target" and even "on target" toxicity may translate into new therapeutic opportunities; thus, toxicology biomarkers should be viewed as potential efficacy biomarkers in select cases, creating an opportunity to build considerable value in molecular targeted approaches.

Overall, while biomarker-guided development is quickly becoming a powerful and necessary tool in support of development of innovative molecular targeted therapies, validation of select biomarkers as diagnostics—although still a lengthy and expensive process—may help expand the clinical and commercial opportunity of a novel drug by directing treatment to patient populations that would benefit the most.

CASE STUDY: TRANSLATIONAL APPROACH APPLIED TO AN INVESTIGATIONAL CANCER VACCINE

Herein, we illustrate the translational concept applied to a new cancer vaccination approach encompassing recombinant DNA vectors (Table 1). The overarching aim, resulting from the prior evidence in animal and man, was to develop a cell-free immunization approach that does not encompass replicating or integrating microbial vectors, yet has a chance to elicit potent antitumor responses. Recombinant DNA vectors in the form of plasmids expressing antigen fragments were an appealing strategy since the potential to elicit a broader range of immune responses encompassing MHC class I–restricted T-cell immunity (6) does not replicate in mammalian cells and does not significantly integrate into the host's genome (7). There are, however, several pitfalls associated with plasmid vectors when used as vaccines: first and foremost, the low magnitude of immune response achieved particularly in humans but also in the preclinical models (the data in preclinical models were overestimated primarily because of availability of highly sensitive assays and inbred species—not applicable to primate situation). Upon considerable effort in outlining the causes, we know now that the major factors responsible for the limited immunogenicity of plasmid vaccines are (1) the low rate of in vivo transfection of resident cells capable to support cross-priming mechanisms or directly prime the T cells and (2) the rapid silencing of the expressed insert, promoter, and/or regulatory elements by host cells' methylation apparatus. Overall, within several tens or hundreds of cells at the injection site this resulted in very low antigen expression that lasted only for several days—despite persistence of inert plasmid for weeks if not months (8). Several key studies demonstrated how important was the limited number of antigen-expressing APCs achieved by plasmid injection in determining the modest immune response (9). For example, adoptive transfer of escalating

Table 1 A Translational Approach in Support of a Novel, Plasmid-Based Active
Immunotherapeutic Strategy (Cancer Vaccine)

Steps (in chronological order)	Rationale	References
Naked plasmid for immunization (intramuscular injection)	Plasmid induces broad immune responses in preclinical models	22
Naked plasmid for intralymphatic immunization	Limited magnitude of immunity by intramuscular immunization	10
Plasmid priming, peptide boost, by intralymphatic administration	Limited magnitude of immune response by plasmid immunization in man	12, 13
	High-quality immune response afforded by plasmid priming	23
	High magnitude of immune response afforded by peptide boost	17
Multitargeted, plasmid priming, peptide boost approach, using intralymphatic immunization	Coexpression of several defined tumor-associated antigens within cancer tissue	18, 19, 24
Biomarker-guided clinical exploration of a prime boost, intranodal immunization approach	Coexpression of target antigens across several tumor types	18, 19, 24
Expanded array of assays in support of clinical exploration of a prime boost, intranodal immunization approach	Evidence that preexisting immunity was associated with improved clinical outcome	13

number of antigen-expressing cells pooled from many animals immunized with
plasmid, resulted in greatly magnified immune responses as compared to those
achieved in animals immunized with the same plasmid (9).

On the basis of such observations and the hypothesis that directly transfected APCs are more potent in inducing immune responses, several preclinical
studies showed that direct intrasplenic or lymphatic injection of plasmid has a
potential to generate superior responses (10). There was significant excitement
generated by the finding that minute amounts of plasmid delivered to the APC-
rich skin by gene gun immunization, or secondary lymphoid tissue, were able to
elicit robust immunity in preclinical models (10,11). A closer look at the data
showed that while less plasmid was required to elicit an immune response, the
overall dose-effect plateau in terms of achievable immune response was not
dramatically changed. Nevertheless, early-phase clinical trials encompassing
plasmid infusion into the groin lymph nodes of patients with advanced melanoma were carried out to test the safety and immunogenicity of this approach
(12,13). For example, a more recent trial encompassed a plasmid-expressing
Melan-A/MART-1 epitopes including the previously characterized HLA-
A2-restricted Melan-A_{26-35} epitope (13). The plasmid was slowly infused into

the groin lymph nodes of 19 melanoma patients with stage IV disease, using a programmable infusion pump. The plasmid was given in repeated cycles, generally up to four times; each cycle lasting 96 hours and being two weeks apart. The trial was a dose-ranging, with maximal dose of 1.5 mg of plasmid per infusion cycle. Plasmid infusion into lymph nodes was well tolerated, with few adverse events mostly local (transient lymphadenopathy) and rare systemic adverse events (mainly fatigue and pyrexia). Only 4 out of 19 patients showed measurable elevation of the immune response as assessed by tetramer assay–based measurement of peptide-specific T cells. Interestingly, other five patients had preexisting immunity against Melan-A and showed no further increase in the frequency of specific T cells. Despite the fact that there was no objective tumor regression in any of the patients treated, there was a significant correlation between clinical outcome in terms of TTP and Melan-A immunity at baseline or after immunization. Patients that developed an immune response in both circumstances had a double TTP than the nonimmune patients. A lack of correlation with the basic immune competency measurements (percentage of $CD4^+$, $CD8^+$ T cells and ex vivo mitogenic test) argued against the possibility of a bias or that Melan-A/MART-1-specific immunity is simply an epiphenomenon (linked to the overall immune competence and thus clinical status). Nevertheless, the statistical significance of this retrospective analysis disappears if patients with preexisting immunity against Melan-A are excluded from the analysis. In the absence of a detailed analysis of the immunological response (for example, the profile of T cells before and after immunization), we cannot rule out that, in fact, despite the lack of further expansion of the antigen-specific population in these patients, the vaccine may have acted by converting the T cells to an effector phenotype. Conversely, only four patients apparently displayed de novo induction of specific immunity against the dominant Melan-A_{26-35} epitope evaluated in this trial.

Overall, the conclusions were the following:

- Melan-A/MART-1 and tyrosinase are most likely key melanoma antigens that offer a viable platform for developing immunotherapies—concordant with independent findings (14).
- The immunization methodology needs significant improvement in order to allow induction of robust, reproducible, persisting, and multivalent immune responses.
- The range and quality of assays in support of the exploratory trials need to be enhanced.
- Evaluation of multiple PD biomarkers in exploratory phase is of paramount importance to development of first-in-class products. Example in case, the need to have a comprehensive evaluation of magnitude and profile of immune response. This is key to establish a causal link between the investigational drug and the clinical effect during early development, a prerequisite for successful identification of the right opportunity in clinic

Antigen
Category
(in non-vaccinated
patients)

Prospective mechanisms of action of
cancer vaccines

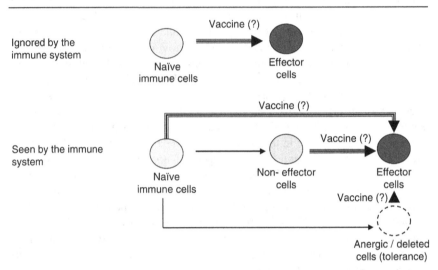

Figure 13 Cancer vaccine design as guided by the immune nature of target antigens.

and the overall success of the program during drug development, and
further, in the marketplace. It is particularly important, for cancer vaccines
in development, to consider this point and take into account the diversity of
prospective mechanisms of action, since there is still much debate on the
significance of preexisting immunity or tolerance relative to the potential
efficiency of vaccination (Fig. 13).

- Implement a biomarker-guided eligibility-criteria approach to maximize
  the opportunity of the investigational drug during the exploratory phase. In
  this case, exclude patients that do not express within the tumor tissue the
  target antigens or do not display a given HLA type and therefore will not
  have any reasonable chance for clinically benefiting, should the pharmacological response be present.

The overarching message is to optimize the approach through exploration before
advancing to randomized efficacy trials (phase 2b) and certainly, confirmatory
pivotal trials used for registration. These conclusions were further used in con-
cordance with a translational approach (bedside to bench) in order to optimize
the investigational drug prior to further development (Fig. 2).

From a mechanistic point of view, the emerging view based on preclinical
and clinical studies is that irrespective of how many APCs are exposed to the

plasmid by various vaccination strategies, there seems to be an intrinsic limitation to overall magnitude of immune response. More recent evidence suggested that the reduced transcriptional competency of transfected APC might be the key limiting factor in this regard. This is also supported by the finding that mRNA-based vectors may be able to circumvent this bottleneck (15). Consequently, simply increasing the transfection of resident cells will not necessarily result in a substantial magnification of the immune response.

One of the methodologies to address the overall poor immunogenicity of plasmids was based on the prime-boost approaches. This methodology was aimed to build on the quality of the response elicited by plasmids but complement them with other vectors that are capable to provide a more optimal antigen exposure. Aside microbial vectors (recombinant viruses or microbes), there are very limited options on what agents can be used as boosters: recombinant proteins, polypeptides, cells, and tumor cell lysates. Peptides represent a unique opportunity in light of targeted intra–lymph node delivery since their known suboptimal pharmacokinetic profile when delivered via more conventional routes. Direct peptide injection into lymph nodes, as shown by preclinical studies, achieves a substantial loading of resident APC and, as a result, robust immunity (16). Consequently, plasmid priming followed by peptide boost resulted in even greater amplification of immunity, retaining the profile of immune response imprinted by plasmid priming and dominated by $CD62L^-$ $CD44^{hi}$ $CD27^{hi}$ T cells capable to produce IFN-γ, TNF-α, MIP1α, and RANTES, externalize CD107α, and produce granzyme B upon antigenic challenge (17). This approach, however, achieves expansion of immune responses only against defined epitopes (one epitope per boosting peptide), but not all epitopes that are encompassed by plasmid inserts. To be effective, this approach needs to target epitopes expressed on a majority of tumor cells, and the methodology elicits "epitope-spreading" associated with progressive broadening of immunity against multiple tumor epitopes and antigens. Currently, there are no reliable experimental means to validate such epitopes in humans; to diminish the risk associated with monoepitope or monovalent approaches, we pursued multicomponent, multivalent approaches—flexible enough to allow mixing and matching of the components fitting the patient's tumor antigen expression profile. On the basis of in depth understanding of the MOA, this is consistent with the principle of personalized or stratified medicine allowing to treat the patients who have the higher likelihood of response. Finally, an expanded array of assays is needed to explore in a comprehensive fashion the pharmacological response and improve on the likelihood of correlating aspects of the biological response with clinical outcome, as well as establish a cause-effect relationship between the investigational drug and clinical effect. This latter aspect is key to directing subsequent development of cancer vaccines in addition to providing decisional flexibility based on solid data sets.

Overall, this translated into two optimized, multicomponent, investigational drugs that are either in clinical trials (18,19) or in the last preclinical development stages (Fig. 14). The peptide analogues used as boosting agents

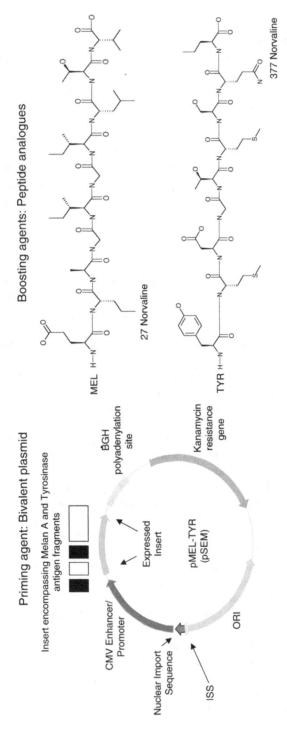

Figure 14 (*See color insert.*) Schematic representation of a multicomponent investigational agent encompassing a plasmid vector and two peptide analogues.

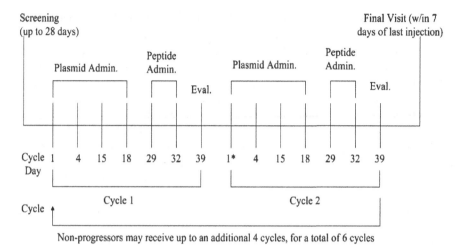

Non-progressors may receive up to an additional 4 cycles, for a total of 6 cycles

* Day 1 of Cycle 2 begins on Day 43

Figure 15 Diagram summarizing a clinical trial designed to evaluate safety and pharmacological response to a biomarker-guided investigational cancer vaccine.

encompass substituted amino acids at primary MHC anchor residues, achieving an increased MHC-peptide half-life and consequently immunogenicity (18–20). Finally, the clinical trial design encompasses the biomarker-guided approach principle with a screening interval for evaluation of HLA and tumor antigen expression, followed by repeat prime-boost cycles as long as the patients do not progress under treatment and regular sample harvesting for comprehensive evaluation of biological response (Fig. 15).

ADAPTIVE TRIAL DESIGNS IN EXPLORATORY PHASE

One of the most interesting aspects characterizing the drug development process once it enters clinic is the antagonism between the speed of executing the clinical trials and budget constrains—a hallmark of the biopharmaceutical business prior to reaching proof of concept in man. This is particularly acute for investigational drugs that are first in class or truly innovative technologies. There are two categories of mistakes that plague early drug development in such circumstances. The first one is underestimating the need to thoroughly explore a new technology in clinic prior to randomized trials. This may result in an inadvertent design of key trials prior to optimizing the approach or defining the best opportunity in clinic. An extreme case of this scenario is stopping the development of a potentially viable drug without the appropriate data set to support it (e.g., failing to demonstrate achievement of a secondary clinical end point in a given indication without rigorous evaluation of "on-target" pharmacological effect that may have opened avenues toward alternate indications).

Conversely, a second mistake consists in protracted clinical exploration of a technology that failed to meet key requirements in terms of expected pharmacological effects; again, in an extreme case, this may be due to simply not setting up certain minimal expectations in terms of on-target pharmacological effects or similar end points. In the case of investigational drugs that are first in class, the only benchmark may be represented by nonclinical exploratory data. Therefore, a key prerequisite for successful translation of a new technology or investigational drug is an appropriate design of the clinical exploratory program—a responsibility shared by a variety of departments such as research, development, clinical, operations, and regulatory.

In addition to unavoidable hurdles associated with translating innovative technologies, an additional factor that needs to be taken into account is the molecular targeting nature of new investigational drugs. Therefore, the R&D process starts with the molecular target and there is very limited evidence on its applicability in terms of therapeutic approach and indication. Throughout development and once the project matures, both the therapeutic approaches (small molecule versus biomolecule, high throughput screening versus design) as well as indications start to clarify. From a mathematical standpoint, the number of variables and range of options should be kept at a higher end at the beginning, and will only narrow based on data sets achieved during nonclinical trials and later on based on clinical exploration of both target and investigational drugs. That is quite a different paradigm compared to conventional R&D processes in support of second- and third-generation drugs, where clinical indication at the beginning is a fixed parameter (e.g., new insulins for pulmonary inhalation) (Fig. 15).

To enable a more optimal translational and clinical development of investigational cancer vaccines in an environment devoid of licensed compounds to date, we propose a different clinical exploration paradigm consistent with the basic tenets of translational medicine outlined above. The primary aim of this approach is to generate a relevant data set as early as possible during the clinical exploratory process to appropriately guide the subsequent development. There are several versions of the process that can be imagined to achieve that goal; one of them (Fig. 16) encompasses phase 1/2a trials aimed to test the pharmacological effect at various doses and/or in a variety of tumor types, in addition to confirming the safety profile—the latter with a somewhat diminished yet not abrogated importance. The key feature of this approach is an interim analysis time point when pharmacological response data are analyzed, and on the basis of the information generated, patient accrual continues in select dose/tumor type cohorts in a phase 2a program aimed to expand the pharmacological response data set and complement it with clinical outcome data. The decision to proceed with a narrow range of parameters can be made on lack of meeting preset success criteria at certain doses and/or in various tumor types; therefore, negative

Conventional approach

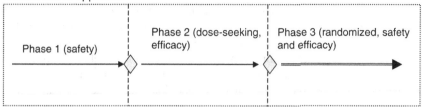

Optimized approach

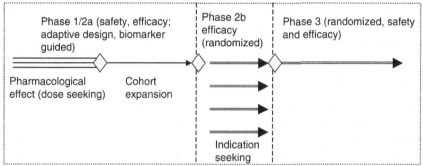

Figure 16 Optimizing the development strategy of cancer vaccines coherent with challenges posed by this class of investigational drugs.

information can be used to narrow down the development process to doses, regimens, and tumor types that are associated with higher likelihood of success. That is provided that preset success criteria were met for one or few of the regimens and/or tumor types. This approach is in line with what has been proposed by a cancer vaccine consortium panel recently (21) and would achieve a considerable amount of information in a shorter interval of time (in addition to safety/toxicity data)—the latter being the major aim of conventional phase 1 trials. The approaches are as follows:

- Definition of dosage/regimens resulting in measurable immune responses;
- Tumor types that have a lower likelihood of supporting immune responses against specific antigens due to various reasons;
- Correlation between immunological response, biomarkers, and clinical outcome; more valuable in phase 2a when the homogeneity of the patient population is higher, after exclusion of less promising tumor types and dosing regimens.

Beyond the phase 1/2a, a phase 2b program would focus on exploring the most promising dosing regimen in several indications associated with one or two tumor types at maximum, via a set of randomized trials carried out in parallel. This approach would achieve a faster evaluation, in an objective fashion, of the efficacy of the cancer vaccine as opposed to using historical controls (a usual source for bias in the case of first–in-class investigational drugs). If used properly, this approach may prevent transition to phase 3 if the drug is not likely to be effective; conversely, this strategy may offer significant information and even anticipate the optimal design of the phase 3 program. In addition, due to the fact that cancer vaccines can be applied as adjuvants in minimal residual disease post-standard therapy, they can be used as a companion to standard therapy (combination approach) or in late stages, in refractory setting as monotherapy. Ideally, all these indications should be explored in parallel in a randomized phase 2b program to provide a data set to make appropriate recommendations for one or multiple pivotal phase 3 trials necessary for defining the product profile and registration.

CONCLUSIONS

In conclusion, due to cancer vaccines' intrinsic nature (targeted therapies with indirect MOA) and scarcity of benchmarks in terms of late-stage or approved products, a re-designed translational approach would be fully beneficial for the development of such therapies. The critical element of this approach is the stratified medicine concept—essentially encompassing biomarker-guided R&D. This approach can be done through an iterative translational strategy aimed to optimize the investigational drug and define the target population prior to randomized trials. In addition, innovative, flexible, and adaptive clinical trial designs will support early generation of relevant data in humans. While there are differences in between technology platforms explored as cancer vaccines, these principles apply irrespectively and should result in an increased likelihood of success. To extract the essence of R&D in the post–human genome project era of molecular targeted approaches, we no longer develop drugs alone but also therapeutic approaches, encompassing both the means to identify the patient and the appropriate medicament.

REFERENCES

1. Gattinoni L, Powell DJ Jr., Rosenberg SA, Restifo NP. Adoptive immunotherapy for cancer: building on success. Nat Rev Immunol 2006; 6(5):383–393.
2. Dudley ME, Wunderlich JR, Robbins PF, et al. Cancer regression and autoimmunity in patients after clonal repopulation with antitumor lymphocytes. Science 2002; 298:850–854.
3. Quezada SA, Peggs KS, Curran MA, et al. CTLA4 blockade and GM-CSF combination immunotherapy alters the intratumor balance of effector and regulatory T cells. J Clin Invest 2006; 116(7):1935–1945.
4. Weber JS, Mulé JJ. How much help does a vaccine-induced T-cell response need? J Clin Invest 2001; 107(5):553–554.

5. Denkberg G, Cohen CJ, Lev A, et al. Direct visualization of distinct T cell epitopes derived from a melanoma tumor-associated antigen by using human recombinant antibodies with MHC-restricted T cell receptor-like specificity. Proc Natl Acad Sci USA 2002; 99(14):9421–9426.

6. Liu MA. The immunologist's grail: vaccines that generate cellular immunity. Proc Natl Acad Sci USA 1997; 94(20):10496–10498.

7. Glenting J, Wessels S. Ensuring safety of DNA vaccines. Microb Cell Fact 2005; 4:26.

8. Coelho-Castelo AAM, Trombone AP, Rosada RS, et al. Tissue distribution of a plasmid DNA encoding Hsp65 gene is dependent on the dose administered through intramuscular delivery. Genet Vaccines Ther 2006; 4:1.

9. Bot A, Stan A.-S., Inaba K., et al. Dendritic cells at a DNA vaccination site express an encoded influenza nucleoprotein and prime CD8+ cytolytic lymphocytes upon adoptive transfer. Int Immunol 2000; 12:825–832.

10. Maloy KJ, Erdmann I, Basch V, et al. Intralymphatic immunization enhances DNA vaccination. Proc Natl Acad Sci USA 2001; 98(6):3299–3303.

11. Fynan EF, Webster RG, Fuller DH, et al. DNA vaccines: protective immunizations by parenteral, mucosal, and gene-gun inoculations. Proc Natl Acad Sci USA 1993; 90(24):11478–11482.

12. Tagawa ST, Lee P, Snively J, et al. Phase I study of intranodal delivery of a plasmid DNA vaccine for patients with Stage IV melanoma. Cancer 2003; 98(1):144–154.

13. Weber J, Boswell W, Smith J, et al. Phase I trial of intranodal injection of a Melan-A/MART-1 DNA plasmid vaccine in patients with stage IV melanoma. J Immunother 2007 (in press).

14. Yee C, Thompson JA, Byrd D, et al. Adoptive T cell therapy using antigen-specific CD8+ T cell clones for the treatment of patients with metastatic melanoma: in vivo persistence, migration, and antitumor effect of transferred T cells. Proc Natl Acad Sci USA 2002; 99:16168–16173.

15. Heiser A, Coleman D, Dannull J, et al. Autologous dendritic cells transfected with prostate-specific antigen RNA stimulate CTL responses against metastatic prostate tumors. J Clin Invest 2002; 109(3):409–417.

16. von Beust BR, Johansen P, Smith KA, et al. Improving the therapeutic index of CpG oligodeoxynucleotides by intralymphatic administration. Eur J Immunol 2005; 35:1869–1876.

17. Smith KA, Qiu Z, Der-Sarkissian A, et al. Immunological Control and Regression of Solid Tumors Achieved by Lymph Node Targeted Immunotherapy. Los Angeles, CA: International Society for Biological Therapy of Cancer, 2006 (J Immunother 2006; 29(6):676–677).

18. Bot A, Qiu Z, Liu L, et al. A novel class of biotherapeutics co-targeting cancer cells and the associated tumor neovasculature. Alexandria, VA: International Society for Biological Therapy of Cancer, 2005 (J Immunother 2005; 28(6):637–638).

19. Smith K, Qiu Z, Tam V, et al. DNA Vaccination Revisited: Induction of Potent Immunity by Sequential Injection of Lymph Nodes with Plasmid Vectors and Peptides. Los Angeles: Annual AACR Meeting, 2007.

20. Busch DH, Pamer EG. MHC class I/peptide stability: implications for immunodominance, in vitro proliferation, and diversity of responding CTL. J Immunol 1998; 160(9):4441–4448.

21. Hoos A, Parmiani G, Hege K, et al. Cancer Vaccine Clinical Trial Working Group. A clinical development paradigm for cancer vaccines and related biologics. J Immunother 1997–2007; 30(1):1–15.

22. Ulmer JB, Donnelly JJ, Parker SE, et al. Heterologous protection against influenza by injection of DNA encoding a viral protein. Science 1993; 259(5102):1745–1749.

23. Roman M, Martin-Orozco E, Goodman JS, et al. Immunostimulatory DNA sequences function as T helper-1-promoting adjuvants. Nat Med 1997; 3(8):849–854.

24. Mashino K, Sadanaga N, Tanaka F, et al. Expression of multiple cancer-testis antigen genes in gastrointestinal and breast carcinomas. Br J Cancer 2001; 85(5): 713–720.

9

Diagnostic Approaches for Selecting Patient-Customized Therapies, Obviating Tumor Variability to Maximize Therapeutic Effect

Chih-Sheng Chiang, Nathalie Kertesz, and Zheng Liu
Division of Translational Medicine, MannKind Corporation, Valencia, California, U.S.A.

NEED FOR DIAGNOSTIC INFORMATION TO GUIDE TARGETED THERAPY (THERANOSTICS)

One of the promising concepts for improving health care utilizing the considerable knowledge gained in the past century is personalized medicine or individualized medicine. Basically, the promise is that therapeutic efficacy can be maximized while minimizing side effects if treatments are designed according to the relevant genotype and phenotype information of the individual (1). Another aspect of personalized medicine is monitoring the evolution of the disease (including the effects of treatment and changes of the disease target itself) and adjusting further therapy accordingly. In order to obtain the relevant information of the individual and monitor the disease evolution, appropriate diagnostic methods need to be applied. Therefore, the approach of utilizing relevant diagnostic information to guide therapy (known as theranostics) has become an essential component of personalized medicine.

Cancer is a very complex collection of diseases. Not only are there multiple organ types and histotypes, but also the underlying molecular variations in each type of cancer are numerous (2,3). Genomic instability has been observed in most types of tumors, and mutations accumulate at accelerated rates in cancer cells. Therefore, cancer of the same type will be different from one patient to the next (4). Moreover, there is considerable heterogeneity within the same type of cancer in a single patient. That is, within the same patient, some cancer cells would have different characteristics from other cancer cells (4).

The limited efficacy and lack of standardization of conventional chemotherapy have lead to the development and implementation of alternative strategies for the treatment of malignant diseases. The role of immune surveillance in the control of tumor growth has sparked a large amount of attention on immunotherapy (5). Another factor that has placed immunotherapy on the forefront of new cancer therapies is the significant progress in the identification of human tumor–associated antigens (6) and in the characterization of the molecular steps leading to an immune response (7).

Immunotherapy of cancer generally targets tumor-associated antigens (TAA) frequently expressed in cancers but seldom in normal tissues. In passive immunotherapy, an immunologically active molecule such as monoclonal antibody is provided by the treatment. Thus, loss or downregulation of target antigen expression by a tumor cell would allow it to escape the immunity generated or provided by immunotherapy.

In active immunotherapy, a substance capable of inducing the patients' own immunity to the targeted antigens is provided by the treatment. The emphasis has been on T cell–based immunotherapy, because T cells, especially cytolytic T cells (CTL), are generally believed to play a major role in the control of tumor growth (8). Antigen-specific CTL recognize specific human leukocyte antigen class I (HLA1)-TAA–derived peptide complexes on the cell surface. These complexes are generated, transported to the cell membrane, and presented to CTL through a series of sequential steps including proteasomal cleavage of proteins in the cytoplasm (9), transport of peptides by the transporter associated with antigen-processing complex (TAP1-TAP2) to the endoplasmic reticulum (10), and loading of peptides on the β_2-microglobulin (β_2M)–HLA1 heavy chain complex (11,12). The peptide-β_2M-HLA1 heavy chain complex then travels to the cell membrane and is presented to CTL.

In the last decade, there has been renewed interest in the class I major histocompatibility complex (MHC1) antigens in tumors with the realization of the crucial role played by MHC1 antigens in the recognition of tumor cells by CTL (13) and with the emphasis on T cell–based immunotherapy for the treatment of human cancer (14,15). Most MHC1-presented peptides are derived from endogenous proteins such as tumor antigens and viral antigens. Approximately 40–90% of human tumors derived from various MHC1-positive tissues were reported to be MHC1 deficient. Furthermore, tumor cells with downregulated MHC1 antigen expression show enhanced growth and are frequently associated

Table 1 Benefits of Patient Stratification for Immunotherapy

Improve response rate
Obviate tumor variability
Maximize treatment efficacy
Minimize adverse side effects
Avoid unnecessary exposure to therapeutic agents
Save valuable time and health-care money

with disease progression toward the invasive and metastatic tumor phenotype (16). Abnormalities in the expression and/or function of antigen-processing machinery components and/or HLA1 may lead to defects in the expression of HLA1-peptide complexes and defects in the recognition of targets by CTL. This seems to be used as an escape mechanism by tumor cells to escape from immune recognition and destruction (17). Additionally, production of factors that block effector cell functions locally would also enable the cancer cell to become resistant to the immune response induced by the therapy (18) and may account for the unexpected poor prognosis of the disease in patients with high expression of HLA1 in primary and/or metastatic lesions (19) and with recurrence of the disease in patients treated with T cell–based immunotherapy (20,21). Therefore, patient stratification or selection before prescribing immunotherapy is necessary for achieving the best efficacy and for minimizing undesirable side effects. From an economic point of view, it is also important to select the patient population most likely to benefit from the therapy so that health-care money is spent effectively (Table 1).

APPROACHES TO IMPROVE EFFICACY FOR IMMUNOTHERAPY AND MINIMIZE PROBLEMS OF TUMOR VARIABILITY

Patient Stratification

Clinical evaluation of targeted cancer therapy is currently limited by the difficulty in matching a new molecularly targeted agent to the appropriate molecular-defined patient. In order to circumvent this difficulty it is important to have patient-positive selection criteria by performing target-based expression screening. It is also important to have assays in place for patient monitoring in order to optimize drug dosage and assess response to treatment. Recent clinical developments, such as the demonstrated antitumor activity of specific monoclonal antibodies (anti-CD20 and anti-Her2/neu), have contributed to renewed enthusiasm in immunotherapy and the acceptance of the need to allow selection of patients eligible for the treatment depending on the expression of the tumor antigens. This has helped oncologists to select patient populations most likely to respond to the treatment. Emerging improvements in technologies are enabling the stratification of cancers, the ability to follow cancer progression, the ability to stratify patients as responders or non-responders to therapy, and the ability to monitor *in vivo* cancer biology and therapeutic responses.

Demonstrating the presence of targeted antigens in cancer cells is an important first step for selecting patients most likely to respond. A number of methods have been used to demonstrate that the targeted antigens are present in the cancer cells. The methods include traditional methods such as immuno-histochemistry (IHC) and cytogenetics as well as newer molecular methods such as RTPCR, PCR, and in situ hybridization. PCR and RTPCR are highly sensitive methods; under favorable conditions, the presence of a few molecules of nucleic acids in the sample can be detected. However, these methods lack the ability to indicate the spatial distribution of the target molecules in reference to morphological features. For example, the detection of PSMA mRNA in a tumor sample cannot indicate whether PSMA is expressed by the tumor cells or neovasculature surrounding the tumor cells. Furthermore, the detection or quantitation of mRNA would not provide direct information on the amount of the protein antigen in tumor cells or its subcellular location. In addition, the detection of mRNA in formalin-fixed paraffin-embedded (FFPE) tumor samples (the most common type of archived samples) is difficult because of RNA degradation during the processing steps and storage of the FFPE samples (Table 2).

IHC (and other in situ techniques), though potentially more labor intensive, allow spatial variation of expression within a sample to be observed. Distinctions can be made such as coexpression of antigens within the same cells providing for greater redundancy of targeting and reduced likelihood of escape mutants arising by antigen loss, and coexpression within different cells within the same sample, revealing how a greater proportion of the total tumor tissue can be directly targeted. Such information is also relevant to the use of antigens with more complex expression patterns. For example, PSMA, which can be expressed by

Table 2 Assays for Patient Stratification in Targeted Immunotherapies

Name	Use
IHC	Ascertain tumor tissue expresses targeted antigen
RTPCR	Ascertain tumor tissue expresses targeted antigen
Immune competence[a]	Ascertain patients' immune function
HLA genotyping[b]	Make sure patient has targeted HLA type
Flow cytometry[c]	Ascertain tumor cells expresses targeted antigen

[a]for active immunotherapies only.
[b]for T-cell–based active immunotherapies and passive immunotherapies relying on presence of HLA-peptide epitope complexes.
[c]for leukemia.

prostate cells and tumor neovasculature, can be used as a prostate lineage marker if its expression can be associated specifically with the neoplastic cells through use of an *in situ* detection methodology.

For active immunotherapies, an assessment of the patient's immune competence would also be appropriate. Commonly used tests include delayed hypersensitivity, *in vitro* lymphocyte proliferation, among others. Additionally, the presence of HLA and accessory molecules in cancer cells would be needed for active immunotherapies that rely on cytolytic T cell responses. T cell receptor–like antibodies (TCRL Ab) are antibodies that bind specifically to a particular peptide-HLA1 complex, but not the peptide by itself or the HLA1 molecule complexed with other peptides. This binding is in a manner similar to T-cell receptors (TCRs). TCRL Ab can be used for detecting the presence of peptide-HLA1 complexes on the tumor cell surface.

Response Monitoring

After the therapy is given, monitoring the response of the patient is important. In addition to clinical parameters, monitoring changes of the targeted antigen in the cancer cells would be important. If a patient's tumor initially regressed but relapses after some period of time, analyzing the cancer cells at time of relapse would be useful, if appropriate specimens can be obtained. The information obtained at time of relapse would provide the basis for considering another form of therapy or similar therapy targeting another antigen. For example, if mutations in the targeted antigen were detected, then similar therapy targeting a different antigen may be considered. However, if HLA expression of the cancer cells was lost, then therapies that depend on CTL would not be appropriate (Table 3).

For active immunotherapies, monitoring of the patient's immune response to the targeted antigen will provide a fast glimpse of the effect of therapy. For patients who do not mount a significant immune response to therapy, it may be appropriate to consider changing the treatment. This would save precious time for potentially more efficacious treatment without waiting until clinical response is manifest (Table 4).

Thus, monitoring patients' response after initiation of therapy will provide useful information needed for considering and guiding further therapy.

Table 3 Benefits of Monitoring Response to Treatment

Objective information as basis for modifying therapy or selecting new therapies
Timely stop of ineffective treatment minimizes exposure to ineffective
   treatment and its undesirable side effects
Early commencement of alternative therapies saves valuable time and money

Table 4 Assays for Monitoring Patients' Immune Response

Name	Use
Antibody titer	Detect patients' humoral immune response to targeted antigen
Tetramer	Measure magnitude of patients' specific T-cell response to targeted antigen
ELISPOT	Measure magnitude and function of patients' specific T-cell response to targeted antigen
Flow cytometry of T-cell markers	Assess T-cell response to targeted antigen as measured by expression of relevant cytokines or other markers

EXAMPLES

Using Diagnostic Assays in Pretreatment Screening and Eligibility Criteria

IHC of TAA and HLA Marker (β_2M)

The fact that human cancer cells express antigens has been directly addressed by the identification and cloning of a number of tumor-associated and tumor-specific antigens. MKC has focused on TAA-specific antigens that are highly expressed in many different cancers including prostate, breast, ovarian, pancreatic, renal cell, colorectal carcinomas, and melanoma. MKC has assays in place for determining the patient's MHC1 type for HLA-A2 specificity, assaying the patient's tumor tissue for two or more expressed target TAAs, assaying the patient's tumor tissue for the expression of β_2M, and selection of the correct immunotherapeutic targets for administration to the patient based on the assays. Our preselected panel of TAAs includes cancer testis antigens, tissue-specific antigens, differentiation antigens, and lineage-specific markers. The targets comprise two or more antigens: PSMA, PRAME, Tyrosinase, Melan-A/MART-1, and NY-ESO-1, SSX-2. Our TAA targets are expressed by the tumor cell as well as in the tumor-associated neovasculature or stroma in primary tumor tissue or metastatic tumors. With our assays, antigen expression can be detected, directly or indirectly by detection of the absence, presence, and/or abundance of mRNA, polypeptide, mature protein, peptide, or MHC-peptide complex. All the assays we have in place detect the condition of the TAAs as well, such as processing state, differential splicing, mutation from germline, variation from consensus sequence in human population, cellular localization, subcellular localization, coexpression with other markers, and the like. Examples include reverse transcription polymerase chain reaction (RT-PCR), real-time PCR, quantitative PCR, northern hybridization, autoradiography, chemiluminescent detection, autofluorography, flow cytometry, gene chip expression profiling, IHC, western blot, radioimmunoassay (RIA), or *in situ* hybridization, individually or in any combination thereof. At least two assaying steps are carried out at different time points during the course of disease, and comparative information is obtained from the assaying steps. The obtained information can be used to help decide how and when to implement, modify, or withdraw a therapy. PCR techniques are sensitive and generally easy to implement; however, they cannot detect the mosaicism of antigen expression within a sample. IHC (and other in situ techniques) provides the means to observe the spatial variation of expression.

Antibody-based techniques can offer the advantage of directly detecting protein expression at the cell surface, which is of clinical relevance, in contrast to RT-PCR and the like, from which surface expression can only be inferred. In general, immunohistochemical staining allows the visualization of antigens via the sequential application of a specific antibody (primary antibody) that binds to the antigen, a secondary antibody that binds to the primary antibody, an enzyme complex, and a chromogenic substrate with washing steps in between. The enzymatic activation of the chromogen results in a visible reaction product at the antigen site. The specimen may then be counterstained and cover slipped. Results are interpreted using a light microscope and aid in the differential diagnosis of pathophysiological processes, which may or may not be associated with a particular antigen. Over the past two decades, the availability of HLA-specific monoclonal antibodies (mAb) suitable for immunohistochemical staining and technical advancements in immunohistochemical staining techniques have allowed extensive analysis of HLA1 expression, HLA-specific markers, such as $\beta_2 M$, and TAA. However, suitable antibodies for the IHC detection of type-specific HLA1 molecules in FFPE samples remained difficult to obtain. We have generated highly specific monoclonal antibodies that are peptide specific by Hybridoma technology, in house for two of our target TAA, Prame and SSX2. Antibodies for PSMA, Melan-A, Tyrosinase, and NY-ESO-1 are available commercially.

The expression of polymorphic determinants of HLA1 requires the association of HLA1 heavy chains with $\beta_2 M$. Therefore, class I expression can be assessed by detection of $\beta_2 M$. To this end, sections of formalin-fixed lesions are stained with mAb recognizing $\beta_2 M$ in immunoperoxidase reactions. The $\beta_2 M$ protein is a component of the MHC1. Humans synthesize three different types of class I molecules designated HLA-A, HLA-B, and HLA-C. These differ only in their heavy chain, all sharing the same type of $\beta_2 M$, which is highly conserved. MHC1 is formed by the association of $\beta_2 M$ and an alpha protein, heavy chain, which comprises three domains: $\alpha 1$, $\alpha 2$, and $\alpha 3$. $\beta_2 M$ associates with the $\alpha 3$ subdomain of the α heavy chain and forms an immunoglobulin domain-like structure that mediates proper folding and expression of MHC1 molecules. MHC1 is found on the surface of most types of nucleated cells, where it presents antigens derived from proteins synthesized in the cytosol to $CD8^+$ T cells. Two signals are required for activation of naive $CD8^+$ T cells, the first provided by the interaction of the TCR with the MHC1-antigen complex on the antigen-presenting cell (APC) surface, and the second, costimulation, generated by the interaction of a ligand on the costimulatory APC with a second receptor present on the T-cell surface. The best characterized costimulatory molecules on APCs are the structurally related glycoproteins B7.1 (CD80) and B7.2 (CD86), which interact with the CD28 receptor on the T-cell surface. Activation of CD8$^+$ T cells by these two signals leads to the proliferation of antigen-specific cytotoxic T cells (CTLs), which recognize and destroy cells presenting the signaling antigen. The immunotherapeutic agent induces a T-cell response, especially including a MHC1-restricted T-cell response. Thus, it can be advantageous to confirm MHC expression by the tumor tissue. Reagents for detection of MHC, including for PCR and antibody-based methods, are widely available. Class-, locus-, and type-specific reagents are in common usage. The advantage of having class- and locus-specific reagents allows for a broadly applicable uniform procedure. Type-specific reagents allow for simultaneous confirmation of expression and MHC type.

Multi-analyte IHC

Because the biology of cancer is complicated, many predictive biomarkers must be combined in panels to improve accuracy. Immunohistochemical assays are well reimbursed by Medicare and insurance and accepted by pathologists and oncologists, but only detect one protein at a time. It is often useful to be able to stain for two or more antigens in one common tissue section. This can be achieved by immunofluorescence method using different fluorescent dyes. Multiple staining can also be done with peroxidase-conjugated antibodies developed with different chromogen substrates to produce the end products of different colors. Multi-analyte IHC has the benefit of providing more information on the same specimen, preserving precious clinical material, and allowing for cell subtyping prior to analysis. All multiplex fluorescence techniques rely on the ability of the detection apparatus to separate the light emitted by different fluorescent dyes that label the specimen. Unfortunately, the emission spectra of most fluorophores are broad so that when multiple fluorophores are used together, their emission spectra are difficult to deconvolute. Innovations in microscopy hardware and software partly address the problem of spectral overlap. Linear unmixing has been implemented in the latest generation of confocal microscopes from Zeiss (LSM510-META), allowing the separation of multiple fluorophores. However, when dealing with certain tissue, endogenous autofluorescence contributes to a shift of the spectrum peak from different fluorophores and affects the reliability of linear unmixing when using organic fluorophores. Multi-analyte IHC now makes use of Quantum Dot (Qdots) technology. The unique stability and spectral properties of Qdots have led to their rapid adoption for a variety of molecular-imaging applications. Qdots provide a tool that facilitates the high-throughput multiplex study of gene expression at cellular and subcellular resolution in histological sections. Quantum dots are very small (<10 nm) inorganic fluorophores, made of a semiconductor core that is composed of cadmium sulfide (CdS), cadmium selenide (CdSe), or cadmium telluride (CdTe) and is insulated by a nonreactive ZnS shell and eliminates photon traps. The mixed shell of hydrophobic/philic polymer with carboxylic acid derivatization has a flexible carboxylate surface to which many biological and nonbiological moieties have been attached. The resulting surface can be attached to antibodies, streptavidin, lectins, nucleic acids, and related molecules of biological interest to make them useful for IHC. These novel fluorescent tags have several unique optical properties that make them very suitable for biological applications that require multiplexing and highly sensitive molecular detection. The benefits of quantum immunohistology are that its narrow and symmetric emission reduces cross talk and facilitates multilabeling. Its high photon output and broad absorption spectra make possible the use of a single excitation wavelength that allows for quantitative multiplexing, its high level of brightness and large Stokes shifts help deal with tissue autofluorescence and finally are $100\times$ more resistant to photobleaching than organic dyes and makes them ideal probes for fluorescence quantitation. The slides are stable for long-term archiving. IVD kits are commercially available. By combining this diagnostic product with appropriate analytical software, multi-analyte IHC is a reality. Detection and quantitation of overlapping chromogens accomplished by multispectral imaging is proposed as a tool that can simplify and enrich the extraction of morphological and molecular information. Simple-to-use instrumentation is available that mounts on standard microscopes and can generate spectral image datasets with excellent spatial and spectral resolution; these can be exploited by sophisticated analysis tools. There are commercially available, liquid-crystal tunable-filter-based multispectral imaging platforms. The resulting datasets can be analyzed using spectral unmixing algorithms to separate out the individual dyes and/or learn-by-example classification tools. Multiplexed molecular imaging allows the association of molecular phenotypes with relevant cellular and tissue compartments and conveys new utility to brightfield-based microscopy approaches.

Genotyping HLA

HLA1 molecules are of major importance for antitumor immune responses. Expression of HLA1/β_2M complexes carrying tumor-specific peptides is a prerequisite for adaptively matured CTLs to be able to recognize tumor cells (22). HLA1 are encoded by a family of highly polymorphic genes, with each allele responsible for a different repertoire of antigen presentation. Thus, even the loss of a single allele could potentially allow the escape from an antigen-specific antitumor response. Loss of expression of HLA1 molecules has been frequently reported in a number of malignant lesions (23). Whether these differences reflect technical reasons, patient populations' heterogeneity, and/or the different role played by HLA1 in various types of malignancies is not known. This would therefore represent a serious limitation for vaccine-based antitumor therapies. In the past, the large majority of studies have been performed by immunoperoxidase staining of frozen tissue sections with monoclonal antibodies (mAb) to mono-morphic determinants of HLA1 (24). However, the ease of formalin fixation after surgery required the use of antigen retrieval methods for IHC. Therefore, despite the fact that the use of fresh frozen tissue allows the employment of a higher number of antibodies, complete panels of fresh frozen tissue are not yet readily available. The use of FFPE tissues in immunohistochemical assays was hampered by the very limited availability of anti-HLA1 mAb staining formalin-fixed tissues. To overcome these limitations, mAb recognizing mono-morphic determinants of HLA-A, -B, and -C alleles have been necessary. Still, HLA staining by immunohistochemical analyses (IHC) has a number of intrinsic limitations (25). HLA staining by IHC is often strongly cytoplasmic, which could potentially obscure functionally relevant membranous coex-pression and result in a false negative interpretation. Additionally, an effective tumor immune escape mechanism could occur through a subtle alteration of the tumor cell HLA phenotype. Since the different patterns of HLA1 expression might underlie different tumor behavior and influence the success rate of immunotherapy, it is important to allow for the discrimination of complex phenotypes related to the expression of HLA1. The increased need for accurate HLA typing has led to the use of DNA technology. Molecular typing of the HLA genes has been performed using various techniques that result in different degrees of resolution. This development is reflected by the increase in the number of commercially available kits for HLA1 and HLA2 typing. In addi-tion, new technologies have been created that allow a simple, highly accurate, and rapid approach toward multiplex genotyping of HLA alleles. The PCR–SSOP–Luminex method includes high-throughput, high-resolution genotyping method for the detection of alleles at the HLA-A, -B, -C, and -DRB1 loci by combining PCR and sequence-specific oligonucleotide probes (SSOPs) pro-tocols with the Luminex 100 xMAP flow cytometry dual-laser system to quantitate fluorescently labeled oligonucleotides attached to color-coded microbeads (26). Correct evaluation of genotyping results relies on an up-to-date database. Newly described alleles steadily increase the IMGT/HLA database. The number of alleles has grown steadily since 1968, when fewer than 10 class I alleles were identified and named. By 2007, over 1500 alleles have been identified and named. We have selected the HLA-A*0201 allele as a model for our studies, since this allele has a high frequency in the population, therefore facilitating the recruitment of patients to the study. Furthermore, the HLA-A*0201 allele has been shown to present TAA-derived peptides to CTL (27–29). Lastly, the vast new technology of new DNA-based typing methods that have been developed and are available for the study can provide further means for highly specific and tailored medicine. Besides contributing to and facilitating the screening to determine the antigen expression and HLA typing profiles for patient selection, the outlined studies will generate reagents and methodology that will facilitate the monitoring of patients with malignant diseases to be treated with T cell–based immunotherapy in order to determine the clinical significance and future directions.

It is becoming increasingly advantageous to screen patients for expression of TAA for development of an antigen profile for the tumor in order to select the immunotherapeutic product and/or regimen based on the profile. Besides being advantageous for patient-positive selection for clinical use, these diagnostic methods are also advantageous to determine, diagnose, or confirm diagnosis of cancer and monitoring or predicting disease progression in a cancer patient. The goal is to have an assay in place that is relatively inexpensive to practice and that provides the ability to assay large numbers of samples in a limited amount of time. Tumor tissue to assay can be obtained as bulk tissue through surgery or in cellular form from blood, bone marrow, cellular aspirates, and peritoneal, bronchial, or plural aspirates, among others.

Staining of formalin-fixed tissue sections provides reliable information about the expression of HLA1 in lesions from various types of cancer. The reactivity of anti-HLA1 with various molecular-based technologies and β_2M and TAA mAb with formalin-fixed tissues provides the opportunity to perform retrospective studies, utilizing collections of pathological lesions from patients with detailed information about the clinical course of the disease (30–32). Immunohistochemical analysis of different types of cancer with an apparent different involvement of immunological events in their pathogenesis and in their clinical course generates clinically useful information (32). IHC is broadly applicable, but western hybridization, RIA, and flow cytometry can also be used. Reagents such as T cell lines and hybridomas, and more preferably, antibodies specific for the peptide-MHC complex and TCR tetramers that detect presentation of particular T-cell epitopes from target antigens can also be used (33). TCR tetramer–based assays allow simultaneous confirmation of both MHC and target antigen or target epitope expression and are inherently type specific.

TCR-Like Immunoglobulin (TCRL) as a Potential Diagnostic Tool in Pretreatment Screening

MKC's cancer vaccine is aimed at eliciting an effective CTL response that is the ultimate effector to eradicate tumors. $CD8^+$ T cells recognize tumor cells in an antigen-specific, MHC-restricted manner through the interaction between TCR and a peptide fragment derived from tumor antigens bound to MHC1 molecule. Thus, antigen expression is the prerequisite for patients eligible to receive the vaccine. Despite IHC, RT-PCR, PCR, and in-situ hybridization being the common techniques to address antigen expression, none of them can verify that tumor antigens are processed and presented on MHC1 molecules by tumor cells.

An ideal assay to screen eligible patients for MKC and other vaccine-based strategies for inducing CTL immune responses should be able to directly detect MHC1/peptide complex on the tumor cell surface. Antibodies with TCR-like specificity is essentially a tool for measuring and visualizing such specific MHC complexes on the cell surface. The TCR-like antibodies directed toward epitopes derived from human T cell lymphotropic virus type I (HTLV-1) (34) and tumor antigens have been generated by phage display technique using large human antibody phage library. We have successfully used antibodies with TCR-like specificity to HLA-A2/Tyrosinase$_{369-377}$ in detecting the MHC1/peptide complex on both peptide-loaded JY cells and Tyrosinase-expressing melanoma cell line, Mel 624.38, by flow cytometry as demonstrated in Figure 1. The applicability of TCR-like antibody in IHC is being investigated. The TCR-like antibody is a promising tool to identify patients who might benefit from vaccine treatment.

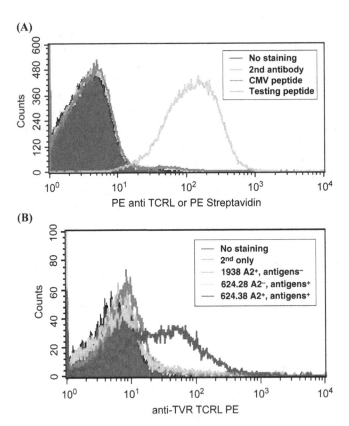

Figure 1 (*See color insert.*) TCR-like antibody against Tyrosinase peptide specifically recognizes Tyrosinase 369–377/HLA-A2 complex on (**A**) peptide-loaded JY cells and (**B**) Tyrosinase expressing, HLA-A2 tumor cell line Mel 624.38.

Immune Response Monitoring as Potential Tool for Therapy Guidance

MKC's cancer vaccine is an active immunotherapy aimed at inducing or augmenting tumor-specific T cells in vivo that leads to tumor regression and survival benefit. With the initiation of various vaccination trials, accurate and reliable assays for testing T-cell function is crucial for the evaluation, comparison, and further development of these approaches. The cellular immune responses have been evaluated using methods measuring cytotoxicity, proliferation, or release of cytokines in a bulk culture. However, these assays often require *in vitro* stimulation prior to performing them. A selection bias is automatically introduced with culturing of the effector cells, and the results subsequently obtained from these assays may not reflect *in vivo* T-cell function.

The emergence of *ex vivo* assays represented by tetramer analysis, ELISPOT assay, and intracellular cytokine staining has significantly improved our ability to measure T-cell response to vaccine attributing to their capability of detecting antigen-specific cell at the single cell level and therefore providing quantitative information. The evolved multiparameter flow cytometry allows us to characterize T-cell subpopulations and provide a better understanding of antitumor immunity.

The immune function varies among individuals, and the variation is amplified among cancer patients. It is common that patients respond to cancer immunotherapy heterogeneously. Therefore, it is important to monitor each individual's immune response to vaccine treatment and adjust the treatment strategy accordingly to achieve clinical benefit. It is logical to measure the increase of tumor-reactive T cells, *in vivo* if any, by tetramer and ELISPOT assays, after vaccine administration. However, recent findings indicate that generation of a large *in vivo* population of tumor-reactive CD8 T cells alone is insufficient to achieve clinically significant tumor regression. Studies applying multiparameter analysis of T-cell phenotypes and functions demonstrate that it is the effective memory response that has a superior antitumor activity (35–37). No doubt, the multiparameter flow cytometry is a valuable addition to tetramer and ELISPOT assay for monitoring immune responses to vaccines.

Tetramer Analysis

The use of MHC1/peptide tetrameric technology to directly visualize and quantify antigen-specific CTLs was first described by Altman et al. in 1996 (38) in which soluble, fluorescently labeled, multimeric MHC/peptide complex bind stably, specifically, and avidly to antigen-specific T cells. This assay is easy to perform; generally 30 minutes staining of tetramer at room temperature is sufficient. Both fresh and cryopreserved PBMC samples have been successfully analyzed and have achieved comparable results (39). The tetramer is able to identify all the T cells specifically recognizing the MHC1/peptide complex composing the tetramer regardless of their functional status. Since the tetramer analysis is a flow cytometry–based assay, it can be used together with other cell surface staining to obtain further characterization of tetramer-positive cells. Alternatively, the tetramer-labeled population can be sorted for additional assays to study its functionality. However, compared with functional assays ELISPOT and intracellular cytokine staining, the sensitivity of the assay is relatively low, and sequences of the antigen epitope peptides have to be available for forming respective tetramers. Some low-affinity clinically important peptide epitopes may not be able to form tetramer efficiently (40). In most cases of immune monitoring, tetramer analysis is accompanied with other functional assays to address functional status of the cells. The immune monitoring workshop in 2002 sponsored by the Society for Biological Therapy recommended that tetramer assay be used in conjunction with ELISPOT or cytokine flow cytometry for evaluating immune responses induced by cancer vaccine (41).

ELISPOT Assay

The ELISPOT assay was originally established to enumerate antibody secreting B cells at the single cell level (42) and later adapted to quantitatively measure the frequency of IFN-γ–producing cells (43). The ELISPOT assay is based on the principle of the ELISA. A 96-well microtiter plate with nitrocellulose or PVDF membrane is coated with a monoclonal antibody against the cytokine of interest. Unseparated PBMCs or isolated $CD8^+$ or $CD4^+$ T cells are incubated with an appropriate antigen for 6–48 hours. In response to recognition of the antigen, cytokine is released by T cells and captured by membrane-bound antibody in the local environment of the cytokine-secreting cells. The cells are washed off and a biotinylated secondary antibody specific to a second epitope of the cytokine is added. To make the antibody-cytokine-antibody sandwich visible, an avidin–enzyme complex and an insoluble enzyme-specific substrate are added. The end result is an area with colored spots, each spot representing a single cell that secretes cytokine.

Similar to ELISA, ELISPOT assay is simple, easy to perform, and amenable to high throughput. This assay is highly sensitive with the reported limit of detection of 1/100,000 (0.001%) compared to 1/10,000 (0.01%) for tetramer analysis (44,45). ELISPOT assay can be performed with either fresh or cryopreserved PBMC samples with similar results (39). However ELISPOT assay is unable to distinguish reactive cell types in polyclonal populations such as PBMCs. Another pitfall of this assay is that each sample can only provide limited information due to the difficulty of multiplexing this assay. How to minimize the operator-dependent variability is another challenge of the assay.

Multiparameter Flow Cytometry

The immune response against the tumor is far more complicated than it was thought before. Not only the magnitude but also the quality of the immune response elicited by the cancer vaccine determines the clinical outcome. The capability of current flow cytometry to measure multiple components of the same samples simultaneously (multiparameter flow cytometry) enables a new biomarker-based approach for monitoring multiple markers of immune responses, which hopefully will be capable of predicting or correlating to clinical effect.

In multiparameter flow cytometry, the antigen-specific T cells are first identified by tetramer or intracellular staining and characterized further by functional and phenotypic markers. The markers of interest include those associated with differentiation and activation status. It has been reported that central memory T cells with the phenotype of $CD45RA^-CCR7^+CD62L^{high}CD27^+$ $CD28^+$ confer superior protective and therapeutic immunity (46–48). $CD107\alpha$, perforin, and granzyme B expression correlates directly with cytotolytic activity of T cells (49). The proliferation capacity can be assessed by CFSE dilutions by flow cytometry (50). In addition to intracellular staining of IFN-γ, accumulation of other cytokines including TNF-α, IL-2, and IL-5, among others can be detected using the same principle (51). Regulatory T cells hallmarked by CD25 and Fox-P3 expression can be identified from a polyclonal population (52). Antigen-specific T cells have to infiltrate the tumor site to exert their antitumor function. Chemokine receptor and adhesion molecule expression on the T-cell surface will predict the possibility of T-cell migration to tumor sites. In a study analyzing chemokine receptor profile of melanoma-specific T cells in patients, the presence of CXCR3 expressing tumor antigen–specific T cells was associated with increased survival (53). The detailed phenotypic and functional analysis of tumor-specific cells and the correlation with clinical response certainly will improve our current understanding of antitumor response and guide development of future immunotherapy strategies.

The multiparameter flow cytometry has been successfully applied in our cancer vaccine preclinical development (54). In the current MKC1106-PP clinical trial, pre- and post-vaccination samples from patients will be analyzed and their phenotype and functionality will be compared.

Use Tetramer and ELISPOT Assay to Monitor Immune Response in Clinical Trial of MKC1106-PP

MKC1106-PP utilizes plasmid prime, peptide boost strategy. Each treatment cycle includes four administrations of plasmid followed by two administrations of peptides. Patients will receive two cycles of vaccination initially. If there is no progression of disease, the patient may receive up to an additional four cycles for a total of six cycles of treatment. To evaluate the efficacy of MKC1106-PP, the immune responses induced by MKC1106-PP will be monitored by both tetramer and ELISPOT assay. The assays will be performed on samples before the treatment, after plasmid priming but before peptide administration, and after peptide boost in each cycle. A substantial increase in the result of tetramer and ELISPOT assays after dosing would indicate that an immune response has been induced in a patient. These two assays have been developed and validated using antigen-specific T cells generated by *in vitro* immunizations.

REGULATORY ISSUES

Regulatory agencies such as FDA (United States Food and Drug Administration) may require that companion diagnostics for selecting patients be available at the time of approval of the immunotherapy. There are several examples such as Herceptin, a monoclonal antibody to Her2/neu, and Her2 diagnostic assays from Dako and Vysis.

FDA issued a Drug-Diagnostic Co-development concept paper in 2005 (Food and Drug Administration 2005, Drug-diagnostic co-development concept paper, draft not for implementation). In the concept paper, the concepts, reasons, and time lines for diagnostic–therapeutic codevelopment were outlined. Since the FDA regulates the diagnostic assay kits, its focus in this paper is on codevelopment of FDA approvable diagnostic kits. A well-known example of codevelopment is the pair of drug-diagnostics Herceptin and HercepTest. Herceptin, a monoclonal antibody against Her2/neu protein, was approved by FDA in 1998 for treating breast tumors overexpressing Her2/neu. At the same time, FDA approved a diagnostic kit, HercepTest, for predicting responsiveness to Herceptin. HercepTest is a kit using immunohistochemical methods for detecting the Her2/neu protein in the tumor cells.

Although specific examples of codevelopment exist (e.g., Herceptin and HercepTest), there is a dearth of clear business models for the industry to follow. The development and validation of a diagnostic test kits require a fair amount of time and money. Getting an FDA approved test kit on the market takes more resources. Therefore, even with the promise of a captive market, it is difficult for a device manufacturer to assume the financial risk to develop a diagnostic test kit and get FDA approval before the market of the therapeutic product is established. Thus, some have turned to developing Clinical Lab Improvement Act (CLIA)-compliant tests and offer the companion diagnostic tests through clinical laboratories.

Clinical laboratories in the United States are regulated by a set of laws and regulations known as CLIA enforced by CMS (Center for Medicare and Medicaid Services), not FDA. Although the cost of developing CLIA-compliant tests would be considerably lower than that of FDA-approved test kits, significant financial liabilities would be incurred. Furthermore, it is unclear how FDA would view the availability of tests in clinical labs as sufficient substitute for FDA-approved kits or reagents and thus adequate for the requirement of companion diagnostics at the time of approval of the therapeutic agent.

For organizations developing targeted immunotherapies, it would be prudent to prepare for companion diagnostics before entering into late-stage clinical trials. Although the proposed guidelines are not finalized yet, we can expect more regulations in this area to come from FDA. According to FDA's concept paper, markers useful for patient stratification should be identified and assays developed during preclinical development phase of the therapeutic product. Tests for stratifying patients suitable for use in a clinical lab should be available before the start of phase 1 trials. If an analytical platform change for testing (e.g., from RIA to EIA) is needed to make the diagnostics more easily adopted by the intended market, the change should be finalized before the start of phase 3 trials so that clinical validation of the test using the new platform can be completed in time.

Different opinions exist for the optimal timing of various activities mentioned in FDA's concept paper, but in general, strategies for satisfying FDA's requirement of companion diagnostics should be formulated in the preclinical development phase and finalized during phase 2 trials, if not earlier. Negotiations with potential diagnostics partners should also begin as soon as the strategy is developed. The earlier an organization developing a promising immunotherapy starts the preparation for getting companion diagnostics ready, the more likely it would be able to navigate the approval process for the immunotherapy product without surprises and costly delays.

CONCLUSIONS

It is clear that we are evidencing a rapidly changing situation where more and more diagnostic information will be used before and throughout the treatment period to guide the therapy for cancer. Even for conventional chemotherapeutic agents, relevant biochemical characteristics of cancer cells can be used to select patients before therapy to improve response rates and outcome (55). This trend is also evident in other fields such as infectious diseases. For example, genotyping and phenotyping of HIV have been widely used to guide drug therapy for HIV infection since the 1990s (56). Relevant information of the virus makes rational and efficacious drug combinations possible for the control of HIV infection. Similar pictures are emerging for the treatment of HCV in terms of using genotype information to select the most appropriate drugs for each patient (57).

As we learn more about the mechanisms of pathogenic processes of various diseases and develop more targeted therapies, relevant diagnostic information will be used more frequently to help stratify patients and guide therapy. For example, with the recent demonstration of potentially efficacious agents for ameliorating effects of nonsense mutations (58), use of genotype information (nature of mutation) of the affected gene in diseases such as cystic fibrosis may become essential in the treatment of certain genetic diseases. Therefore, in the next decade, we will probably see more extensive use of diagnostic information to help guide therapies in many diseases in addition to cancer.

Targeted immunotherapies are specific for certain antigens expressed by tumors and hold great promises to improve treatment for many types of cancers where current modalities fall short. However, the exquisite specificity of immunotherapy requires that the targeted antigens be present in the tumor tissue.

Because cancers are very variable, biochemical characteristics of a given type of cancer can differ significantly from patient to patient. Information on the characteristics of the tumor as well as the host will be important for the selection of patients most likely to benefit from immunotherapy. After initiation of immunotherapy, monitoring the host response would allow continuous adjustment of therapy to maximize desired outcome. The combined use of relevant diagnostic information obtained on the cancer tissue as well as that during the course of treatment from individual patients as guidance for therapy would be necessary for maximizing the therapeutic efficacy of immunotherapy (Figure 2).

From a financial vantage point, the same reasoning applies that utilization of relevant diagnostic information will be critical for the most effective use of health-care dollars. Indiscriminate use of specific immunotherapy will increase the cost of health care and may generate undesirable side effects in some patients. From a regulatory point of view, the sooner an organization makes the needed diagnostic tests available, the more likely it would be successful at satisfying FDA requirements for timely approval of its immunotherapy product. Therefore, one should start formulating the strategies for utilizing and developing diagnostic and monitoring assays as early as possible in the development process of an immunotherapeutic agent.

We can obviate tumor variability, maximize the treatment efficacy, minimize adverse side effects, and speed up the approval process of immunotherapeutic drugs if we develop needed tests early and utilize information obtained through testing intelligently.

There is currently an increasingly growing emphasis on genetic testing and individualized therapy to improve drug efficacy and safety with large investments by major pharmaceutical firms in order to provide a competitive advantage. The future holds promise, with the growing availability of analytical capabilities, to perform genome wide association studies during clinical trials enabling the selection of disease susceptibility genes for prognosis, drug discovery, dosing, and selection of therapy and preventative medicine.

There is a significant source of variability observed in the response to drugs, caused by genetic heterogeneity. We could continue to utilize the variability in interethnic and interindividual genetics to facilitate rational drug design and to avoid adverse effects in clinical trials. Thus, one could generate criteria for selecting patients most likely to benefit from a drug without incurring unnecessary risk. The future of theranostics approaches also holds promise for early or preventive therapy that could significantly enhance clinical outcome. Looking farther ahead, the efficacy of administered drugs may be improved, rather than avoiding toxicity as the main objective, by distinguishing good responders from poor responders prior to therapy, changing clinical trial design as we know it. Often, effective drug response is limited to a portion of treated patients, whereas the majority benefits little or not at all. Predicting which patients are most likely to respond best to a particular drug, or which drug will yield optimal effects for a given patient, would represent a significant advance in therapy even with current

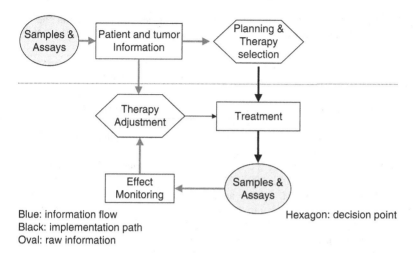

Blue: information flow
Black: implementation path
Oval: raw information

Hexagon: decision point

Figure 2 Theranostic approach.

drugs, let alone novel drugs developed with these criteria in mind. Ultimately this may lead to individualized genetic profiles to select the safest and most effective drug for each individual. The same insight will allow us to achieve the most desirable goal, to prevent disease to begin with.

We are uncertain as to the overall direction of theranostics over the next 10 years. Although new analytical systems introduced during the last decade have offered incremental improvements over previously available technology, there are still many daunting scientific challenges, besides the ethical issues that need to be resolved. Genetic information and individual or ethnic group stratification raises privacy questions and ethical dilemmas about disease susceptibility, prognosis, and treatment options. Obviously, information of this type must be carefully safeguarded to ensure privacy. Many legal and economic issues will need to be resolved. The vision of theranostics is leading us to a more individualized approach to drug therapy, while revealing limits inherent to the treatment of disease in broad patient populations. Whether or not these new technologies and approaches find their way into everyday clinical use during the next 10 years, they will no doubt prove valuable tools in clinical research directed at optimizing drug therapy.

REFERENCES

1. Lesko, LJ. Personalized medicine: elusive dream or imminent reality? Clin Pharmacol Ther 2007; 81(6):807–816.
2. Papadopoulos N, Kinzler KW, Vogelstein B. The role of companion diagnostics in the development and use of mutation-targeted cancer therapies. Nat Biotechnol 2006; 24(8):985–995.

3. Willard HF, Angrist M, Ginsburg GS. Genomic medicine: genetic variation and its impact on the future of health care. Philos Trans R Soc Lond B Biol Sci 2005; 360(1460):1543–1550.

4. Boyer CM, Borowitz MJ, McCarty KS Jr, et al. Heterogeneity of antigen expression in benign and malignant breast and ovarian epithelial cells. Int J Cancer 1989; 43(1): 55–60.

5. Dunn GP, Bruce AT, Ikeda H, et al. Cancer immunoediting: from immuno-surveillance to tumor escape. Nat Immunol 2002; 3(11):991–998.

6. Stevanovic S. Identification of tumour-associated T-cell epitopes for vaccine development. Nat Rev Cancer 2002; 2(7):514–520.

7. Davis ID, Jefford M, Parente P, et al. Rational approaches to human cancer immunotherapy. J Leukoc Biol 2003; 73(1):3–29.

8. Ward PL and Schreiber H. Tumor antigens recognized by T cells. Biological approaches to cancer treatment. Biomodulation. pp. 72–97 (Mitchell, Ed.). New York: McGraw Hill Inc. 1993.

9. York IA, Goldberg AL, Mo XY, et al. Proteolysis and class I major histocompati-bility complex antigen presentation. Immunol Rev 1999; 172:49–66.

10. Lankat-Buttgereit B, Tampé R. The transporter associated with antigen processing: function and implications in human diseases. Physiol Rev 2002; 82(1):187–204.

11. Bouvier M. Accessory proteins and the assembly of human class I MHC molecules: a molecular and structural perspective. Mol Immunol 2003; 39(12):697–706.

12. Momburg F, Tan P. Tapasin-the keystone of the loading complex optimizing peptide binding by MHC class I molecules in the endoplasmic reticulum. Mol Immunol 2002; 39(3–4):217–233.

13. Hicklin DJ, Wang Z, Arienti F, et al. beta2-Microglobulin mutations, HLA class I antigen loss, and tumor progression in melanoma. J Clin Invest 1998; 101(12): 2720–2729.

14. Boon T, Cerottini JC, Van den Eynde B, et al. Tumor antigens recognized by T lymphocytes. Annu Rev Immunol 1994; 12:337–365.

15. Rosenbery SA. Development of cancer immunotherapies based on identification of the genes encoding cancer regression antigens. J Natl Cancer Inst 1996; 88(22): 1635–1644.

16. Benitez R, Godelaine D, Lopez-Nevot MA, et al. Mutations of the beta2-micro-globulin gene result in a lack of HLA class I molecules on melanoma cells of two patients immunized with MAGE peptides. Tissue Antigens 1998; 52(6):520–529.

17. Seliger B, Maeurer MJ, Ferrone S. Antigen-processing machinery breakdown and tumor growth. Immunol Today 2000; 21(9):455–464.

18. Ahmad M, Rees RC, Ali SA. Escape from immunotherapy: possible mechanisms that influence tumor regression/progression. Cancer Immunol Immunother 2004; 53(10): 844–854.

19. van Duinen SG, Ruiter DJ, Broecker EB, et al. Level of HLA antigens in locore-gional metastases and clinical course of the disease in patients with melanoma. Cancer Res 1988; 48(4):1019–1025.

20. Restifo NP, Marincola FM, Kawakami Y, et al. Loss of functional beta 2-micro-globulin in metastatic melanomas from five patients receiving immunotherapy. J Natl Cancer Inst 1996; 88(2):100–108.

21. Jäger E, Ringhoffer M, Altmannsberger M, et al. Immunoselection in vivo: inde-pendent loss of MHC class I and melanocyte differentiation antigen expression in metastatic melanoma. Int J Cancer 1997; 71(2):142–147.

22. Townsend A, Bodmer H. Antigen recognition by class I-restricted T lymphocytes. Annu Rev Immunol 1989; 7:601–624.

23. Hicklin DJ, Marincola FM, Ferrone S. HLA class I antigen downregulation in human cancers: T-cell immunotherapy revives an old story. Mol Med Today 1999; 5(4): 178–186.

24. Marincola FM, Jaffee EM, Hicklin DJ, et al. Escape of human solid tumors from T-cell recognition: molecular mechanisms and functional significance. Adv Immunol 2000; 74:181–273.

25. Leong AS. Pitfalls in diagnostic immunohistology. Adv Anat Pathol 2004; 11(2): 86–93.

26. Itoh Y, Mizuki N, Shimada T, et al. High-throughput DNA typing of HLA-A, -B, -C, and -DRB1 loci by a PCR-SSOP-Luminex method in the Japanese population. Immunogenetics 2005; 57(10):717–729.

27. Crowley NJ, Darrow TL, Quinn-Allen MA, et al. MHC-restricted recognition of autologous melanoma by tumor-specific cytotoxic T cells. Evidence for restriction by a dominant HLA-A allele. J Immunol 1991; 146(5):1692–1699.

28. Kawakami Y, Zakut R, Topalian SL, et al. Shared human melanoma antigens. Recognition by tumor-infiltrating lymphocytes in HLA-A2.1-transfected melanomas. J Immunol 1992; 148(2):638–643.

29. Anichini A, Maccalli C, Mortarini R, et al. Melanoma cells and normal melanocytes share antigens recognized by HLA-A2-restricted cytotoxic T cell clones from melanoma patients. J Exp Med 1993; 177(4):989–998.

30. Natali PG, Nicotra MR, Bigotti A, et al. Selective changes in expression of HLA class I polymorphic determinants in human solid tumors. Proc Natl Acad Sci U S A 1989; 86(17):6719–6723.

31. Kageshita T, Wang Z, Calorini L, et al. Selective loss of human leukocyte class I allospecificities and staining of melanoma cells by monoclonal antibodies recognizing monomorphic determinants of class I human leukocyte antigens. Cancer Res 1993; 53(14):3349–3354.

32. Marincola FM, Ettinghausen S, Cohen PA, et al. Treatment of established lung metastases with tumor-infiltrating lymphocytes derived from a poorly immunogenic tumor engineered to secrete human TNF-alpha. J Immunol 1994; 152(7):3500–3513.

33. Li Y, Moysey R, Molloy PE, et al. Directed evolution of human T-cell receptors with picomolar affinities by phage display. Nat Biotechnol 2005; 23(3):349–354.

34. Cohen CJ, Sarig O, Yamano Y, et al. Direct phenotypic analysis of human MHC class I antigen presentation: visualization, quantitation, and in situ detection of human viral epitopes using peptide-specific, MHC-restricted human recombinant antibodies. J Immunol 2003; 170(8):4349–4361.

35. Rosenberg SA, Sherry RM, Morton KE, et al. Tumor progression can occur despite the induction of very high levels of self/tumor antigen-specific CD8+ T cells in patients with melanoma. J Immunol 2005; 175(9):6169–6176.

36. Speiser DE, Romero P, et al. Toward improved immunocompetence of adoptively transferred CD8+ T cells. J Clin Invest 2005; 115(6):1467–1469.

37. Ayyoub M, Zippelius A, Pittet MJ, et al. Activation of human melanoma reactive CD8+ T cells by vaccination with an immunogenic peptide analog derived from Melan-A/melanoma antigen recognized by T cells-1. Clin Cancer Res 2003; 9(2): 669–677.

38. Altman JD, Moss PA, Goulder PJ, et al. Phenotypic analysis of antigen-specific T lymphocytes. Science 1996; 274(5284):94–96.

39. Maecker HT, Moon J, Bhatia S, et al. Impact of cryopreservation on tetramer, cytokine flow cytometry, and ELISPOT. BMC Immunol 2005; 6:17.

40. Anderton SM, Radu CG, Lowrey PA, et al. Negative selection during the peripheral immune response to antigen. J Exp Med 2001; 193(1):1–11.

41. Keilholz U, Weber J, Finke JH, et al. Immunologic monitoring of cancer vaccine therapy: results of a workshop sponsored by the Society for Biological Therapy. J Immunother (1997) 2002; 25(2):97–138.

42. Czerkinsky CC, Nilsson LA, Nygren H, et al. A solid-phase enzyme-linked immunospot (ELISPOT) assay for enumeration of specific antibody-secreting cells. J Immunol Methods 1983; 65(1–2):109–121.

43. Czerkinsky CC, Tarkowski A, Nilsson LA, et al. Reverse enzyme-linked immunospot assay (RELISPOT) for the detection of cells secreting immunoreactive substances. J Immunol Methods 1984; 72(2):489–496.

44. Asai T, Storkus WJ, Whiteside TL. Evaluation of the modified ELISPOT assay for gamma interferon production in cancer patients receiving antitumor vaccines. Clin Diagn Lab Immunol 2000; 7(2):145–154.

45. Maecker HT, Auffermann-Gretzinger S, Nomura LE, et al. Detection of CD4 T-cell responses to a tumor vaccine by cytokine flow cytometry. Clin Cancer Res 2001; 7(suppl 3):902s–908s.

46. Wills MR, Okecha G, Weekes MP, et al. Identification of naive or antigen-experienced human CD8(+) T cells by expression of costimulation and chemokine receptors: analysis of the human cytomegalovirus-specific CD8(+) T cell response. J Immunol 2002; 168(11):5455–5464.

47. Klebanoff CA, Gattinoni L, Restifo NP. CD8+ T-cell memory in tumor immunology and immunotherapy. Immunol Rev 2006; 211:214–224.

48. Hinrichs CS, Gattinoni L, Restifo NP. Programming CD8+ T cells for effective immunotherapy. Curr Opin Immunol 2006; 18(3):363–370.

49. Betts MR, Brenchley JM, Price DA, et al. Sensitive and viable identification of antigen-specific CD8+ T cells by a flow cytometric assay for degranulation. J Immunol Methods 2003; 281(1–2):65–78.

50. Mannering SI, Morris JS, Jensen KP, et al. A sensitive method for detecting proliferation of rare autoantigen-specific human T cells. J Immunol Methods 2003; 283(1–2):173–183.

51. Suni MA, Picker LJ, Maino VC. Detection of antigen-specific T cell cytokine expression in whole blood by flow cytometry. J Immunol Methods 1998; 212(1):89–98.

52. Graca L. New tools to identify regulatory T cells. Eur J Immunol 2005; 35(6):1678–1680.

53. Mullins IM, Slingluff CL, Lee JK, et al. CXC chemokine receptor 3 expression by activated CD8+ T cells is associated with survival in melanoma patients with stage III disease. Cancer Res 2004; 64(21):7697–7701.

54. Smith KA, Tam V, Qiu Z. Multivalent cellular immune responses detected with iTag™ MHC class I tetramers. Cellular Res 2007; 1:4–5.

55. Ugurel S, Schadendorf D, Pföhler C, et al. In vitro drug sensitivity predicts response and survival after individualized sensitivity-directed chemotherapy in metastatic

melanoma: a multicenter phase II trial of the Dermatologic Cooperative Oncology Group Clin Cancer Res 2006; 12(18):5454–5463.

56. Haubrich R, Demeter L. International perspectives on antiretroviral resistance. Clinical utility of resistance testing: retrospective and prospective data supporting use and current recommendations. J Acquir Immune Defic Syndr 2001; 26(suppl 1): S51–S59.

57. Podzorski RP. Molecular testing in the diagnosis and management of hepatitis C virus infection. Arch Pathol Lab Med 2002; 126(3):285–290.

58. Welch EM, Barton ER, Zhuo J, et al. PTC124 targets genetic disorders caused by nonsense mutations. Nature 2007; 447(7140):87–91.

Index

Printed in the United States
by Baker & Taylor Publisher Services